Recurrent Pregnancy Loss

Recurrent Pregnancy Loss

EDITED BY

Ole B. Christiansen

Unit for Recurrent Miscarriage
Fertility Clinic 4071
Rigshospitalet
Copenhagen, Denmark; and
Department of Obstetrics and Gynaecology
Aalborg University Hospital
Aalborg, Denmark

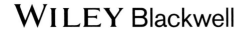

Library of Congress Cataloging-in-Publication Data

Recurrent pregnancy loss / edited by Ole B. Christiansen.
    p. ; cm.–(Gynecology in practice)
  Includes bibliographical references and index.
   ISBN 978-0-470-67294-5 (pbk. : alk. paper) – ISBN 978-1-118-74901-2 –
ISBN 978-1-118-74903-6 (eMobi) – ISBN 978-1-118-74918-0 (ePub) – ISBN 978-1-118-74932-6 (ePdf)
I. Christiansen, Ole B., editor of compilation.   II. Series: Gynecology in practice.
   [DNLM: 1. Abortion, Habitual–prevention & control.   WQ 225]
   RG648
   618.3′92–dc23
                                          2013017940

A catalogue record for this book is available from the British Library.

Contents

Series Foreword

In recent decades, massive advances in medical science and technology have caused an explosion of information available to the practitioner. In the modern information age, it is not unusual for physicians to have a computer in their offices with the capability of accessing medical databases and literature searches. On the other hand, however, there is always a need for concise, readable, and highly practicable written resources. The purpose of this series is to fulfill this need in the field of gynecology.

The *Gynecology in Practice* series aims to present practical clinical guidance on effective patient care for the busy gynecologist. The goal of each volume is to provide an evidence-based approach for specific gynecologic problems. "Evidence at a glance" features in the text provide summaries of key trials or landmark papers that guide practice, and a selected bibliography at the end of each chapter provides a springboard for deeper reading. Even with a practical approach, it is important to review the crucial basic science necessary for effective diagnosis and management. This is reinforced by "Science revisited" boxes that remind readers of crucial anatomic, physiologic, or pharmacologic principles for practice.

Each volume is edited by outstanding international experts who have brought together truly gifted clinicians to address many relevant clinical questions in their chapters. The first volumes in the series are on *Chronic Pelvic Pain*, one of the most challenging problems in gynecology, *Disorders of Menstruation, Infertility*, and *Contraception*. These will be followed by volumes on *Sexually Transmitted Diseases, Menopause, Urinary Incontinence, Endoscopic Surgeries*, and *Fibroids*, to name a few. I would like to express my gratitude to all the editors and authors, who, despite their other responsibilities, have contributed their time, effort, and expertise to this series.

Finally, I greatly appreciate the support of the staff at Wiley-Blackwell for their outstanding editorial competence. My special thanks go to Martin Sugden, PhD; without his vision and perseverance, this series would not have come to life. My sincere hope is that this novel and exciting series will serve women and their physicians well, and will be part of the diagnostic and therapeutic armamentarium of practicing gynecologists.

Aydin Arici, MD
Professor, Department of Obstetrics, Gynecology, and Reproductive Sciences
Yale University School of Medicine
New Haven, CT, USA

Contributors

Muhammad A. Akhtar
Clinical Research Fellow, Reproductive Medicine Unit
University Hospitals Coventry and Warwickshire NHS Trust
University of Warwick, Coventry, UK

Adjoa Appiah
Clinical Research Fellow
Early Pregnancy and Gynaecology Assessment Unit
King's College Hospital
London, UK

Juan Balasch
Institute Clínic of Gynecology, Obstetrics and Neonatology
Barcelona, Spain

Ruth Bender Atik
National Director
The Miscarriage Association
Wakefield, UK

Emmy van den Boogaard
Center for Reproductive Medicine
Department of Obstetrics and Gynecology
Academic Medical Center
Amsterdam, The Netherlands

Howard J.A. Carp
Department of Obstetrics and Gynecology
Sheba Medical Center
Tel Hashomer & Tel Aviv University
Tel Hashomer, Israel

Ricard Cervera
Department of Autoimmune Diseases
Institute Clínic of Medicine and Dermatology
Hospital Clínic
Barcelona, Spain

Ole B. Christiansen
Professor, Unit for Recurrent Miscarriage
Fertility Clinic 4071
Rigshospitalet
Copenhagen, Denmark; and
Department of Obstetrics and Gynaecology

Aalborg University Hospital
Aalborg, Denmark

Silvia Daher
Department of Obstetrics
São Paulo Federal University (UNIFESP)
São Paulo, SP, Brazil

AnnMaria Ellard
Nurse Specialist
Miscarriage Clinic
Liverpool Women's Hospital
Liverpool, UK

Roy G. Farquharson
Gynaecologist
Miscarriage Clinic
Liverpool Women's Hospital
Liverpool, UK

Dida Fleisig
Department of Behavioral Sciences
The College of Management Academic Studies
Rishon Le-Zion, Israel

Mariëtte Goddijn
Center for Reproductive Medicine
Department of Obstetrics and Gynecology
Academic Medical Center
Amsterdam, The Netherlands

Ae-Ra Han
Reproductive Medicine
Department of Obstetrics and Gynecology
Department of Microbiology and Immunology
The Chicago Medical School at Rosalind Franklin University of Medicine and Science
Vernon Hills, IL, USA

Barbara E. Hepworth-Jones
Trustee, The Miscarriage Association
Wakefield, UK

Shehnaaz Jivraj
Consultant Obstetrician and Gynaecologist
Jessop Wing, Sheffield Teaching Hospitals Trust
Honorary Senior Lecturer

University of Sheffield
Sheffield, UK

Jemma Johns
Consultant Obstetrician and Gynecologist
Early Pregnancy and Gynaecology Assessment Unit
King's College Hospital
London, UK

Paulien G. de Jong
Department of Vascular Medicine
Academic Medical Center
Amsterdam, The Netherlands

Claudia Kowalik
Department of Obstetrics and Gynecology
Academic Medical Center
Amsterdam, The Netherlands

Joanne Kwak-Kim
Reproductive Medicine
Department of Obstetrics and Gynecology
Department of Microbiology and Immunology
The Chicago Medical School at Rosalind Franklin University of Medicine and Science
Vernon Hills, IL, USA

Elisabeth C. Larsen
Unit for Recurrent Miscarriage
Fertility Clinic 4071
Rigshospitalet
Copenhagen, Denmark

M. Angeles Martínez-Zamora
Institute Clínic of Gynecology, Obstetrics and Neonatology
Barcelona, Spain

Rosiane Mattar
Department of Obstetrics
São Paulo Federal University (UNIFESP)
São Paulo, SP, Brazil

Saskia Middeldorp
Department of Vascular Medicine
Academic Medical Center
Amsterdam, The Netherlands

Henriette Svarre Nielsen
Department of Obstetrics and Gynaecology
University of Copenhagen
Copenhagen, Denmark

Kuniaki Ota
Reproductive Medicine
Department of Obstetrics and Gynecology
Department of Microbiology and Immunology
The Chicago Medical School at Rosalind Franklin University of Medicine and Science
Vernon Hills, IL, USA

Siobhan Quenby
Professor of Obstetrics
Director of the Biomedical Research Unit in Reproductive Health
Warwick Medical School
University of Warwick, Coventry, UK

Gavin Sacks
Associate Professor, University of New South Wales
St George Hospital
Sydney, NSW, Australia; and
Clinical Director, IVF Australia
Hunter Valley, NSW, Australia

Keren Shakhar
Department of Behavioral Sciences
The College of Management Academic Studies
Rishon Le-Zion, Israel

Maria Regina Torloni
Department of Obstetrics
São Paulo Federal University (UNIFESP)
São Paulo, SP, Brazil

Rosa Vissenberg
Center for Reproductive Medicine
Department of Obstetrics and Gynecology
Academic Medical Center
Amsterdam, The Netherlands

Preface to the First Edition

Recurrent pregnancy loss (RPL), which is almost synonymous with recurrent miscarriage (RM), is defined as a minimum of three (or two) spontaneous losses of intrauterine pregnancies before gestational week 22. It is a cause of involuntary childlessness that among physicians and in the general population is much less recognized than childlessness due to failure to conceive (infertility) or stillbirth. This is mainly due to the fact that whereas there are many established public and private IVF clinics taking care of couples with infertility, as well as many clinics specialized in obstetrics and fetomaternal medicine that take care of women with stillbirths, most women with RPL are being managed in clinics of general gynecology by physicians who often have their main interest in gynecological surgery. A second reason for the invisibility of RPL is that many patients with very early miscarriages or biochemical pregnancies are not coming into contact with hospitals or gynecologic specialists because they have no need for surgical or medical treatment and therefore remain unknown to the secondary and tertiary health-care system. A third reason for the invisibility of RPL may be that since very few treatment options with documented efficacy exist, few physicians feel motivated to take care of these patients. In my experience, only well-educated psychologically strong patients will be able to mobilize the mental energy required to consult one of the few (often distantly located) clinics that have specialized in RPL management. The majority of RPL patients become stuck in the system because few recognize their problems and even fewer can offer them treatments.

Since only a minority of RPL cases are fully recognized by the secondary and tertiary health-care system, no valid registration of the size of the problem exists. Estimates showing that 1% of all women suffer RPL are based on studies conducted 30 years earlier at a time when detecting early pregnancy loss had limited possibilities (no high-resolution vaginal ultrasound, insensitive hCG tests). The real and current prevalence of RPL may be considerably higher than 1% and is also dependent on how the condition is defined: two or more losses versus three or more.

The main goal of this book is to highlight the condition and to help practitioners and gynecologists cope with patients in clinical practice. All chapters are written by specialists who have taken care of patients with RPL in clinical practice and have done recognized research. The reader may be confused by the different opinions put forward by the contributing specialists: some find specific investigations and treatments sufficiently validated to use them or recommend their use in RPL whereas others discourage their use due to limited documentation. In my opinion, this disagreement primarily reflects the fact that there is an urgent need for further specialization and high-quality research in this area. However, the disagreement also reflects the different conditions under which the specialists meet RPL patients: those from private clinics dependent on charging the patients will often have a more liberal approach to tests and treatments while specialists from public clinics who do not charge patients will typically adhere to a more conservative approach to tests and treatments.

As part of the publisher's *Gynecology in Practice* series, the aim of the book is to provide gynecologists in practice or in training with a clinical guide for use in the office or at the bedside.

Therefore, the contributors of the chapters have been asked to write in a practical and concise tone with few references to facilitate easy readability.

I thank all the authors for contributing excellent chapters covering their areas of expertise and for their efforts to write in the expected practical style. I hope that the book will be helpful for improving the management of RPL in clinical practice and for creating public awareness on this hidden cause of childlessness.

Ole B. Christiansen
Professor, DMSc
Unit for Recurrent Miscarriage
Fertility Clinic 4071, Rigshospitalet, Copenhagen, Denmark
and
Department of Obstetrics and Gynaecology
Aalborg University Hospital, Aalborg, Denmark

Obtaining the Relevant History

Ole B. Christiansen[1,2]

[1]Unit for Recurrent Miscarriage, Fertility Clinic 4071, Rigshospitalet,
Copenhagen, Denmark
[2]Department of Obstetrics and Gynaecology, Aalborg University Hospital,
Aalborg, Denmark

Introduction

In most clinics, patients referred with a diagnosis of recurrent miscarriage (RM)
will normally come to a first consultation with a physician where information about
the reproductive history and other medical information are collected, blood samples
are taken, and other relevant investigations are carried out or planned.

Whereas authors in the area of RM often spend plenty of space in their articles
to list the abundance of investigations undertaken in their clinic: hysteroscopy,
endometrial biopsy, parental or fetal karyotyping, screening for thrombophilia,
autoantibodies and microbiobes in addition to endocrine investigations, they spend
very little space (if any) to describe the stringency and accuracy through which
information has been obtained from the patients themselves or their hospital
records. This reflects the modest emphasis most authors lay on reproductive
and disease history compared with information obtained from other kind of
investigations.

In this chapter, I will review information that we aim to collect at the first consultation at my clinic because we (i) find it important for assessing the spontaneous
prognosis for live birth and (ii) it can often point toward etiological factors before any
results from ultrasonic and laboratory investigations are obtained.

The relevant information achievable from the patients themselves or their case
records can be divided into demographic data, reproductive history, disease
history, and family history. The information should be obtained from both partners but the information concerning the women must be considered the most
important.

Demographic data

The most important demographic data are information about parental age, body
mass index (BMI), lifestyle, social class, and occupational factors in addition to
information about the partner.

Recurrent Pregnancy Loss, First Edition. Edited by Ole B. Christiansen.
© 2014 John Wiley & Sons, Ltd. Published 2014 by John Wiley & Sons, Ltd.

Parental Age

High maternal age is one of the strongest negative prognostic factors known. Maternal age over 41–42 years will be decisive for a conservative treatment approach since the dominant risk factor for miscarriage in this age group is embryonal aneuploidy (especially trisomies), which can only be actively treated by IVF with egg donation. The impact of high paternal age on risk of miscarriage and RM is difficult to study since parental ages are strongly correlated and the only couples that are really informative are those few comprising a young woman and an elderly male. The evidence provided so far suggests that high paternal age per se indeed increases the risk of miscarriage, although much less than high maternal age.

BMI

The patients should be weighted and the height measured at the first consultation to obtain a reliable BMI since both BMI below 20 and over 30 have in some studies been reported to decrease the prognosis for live birth in women in the background population and among RM patients. However, a recent study from my clinic showed that high BMI did not exhibit any impact on subsequent miscarriage rate in RM patients with regular menstrual cycles who can conceive spontaneously. BMI may therefore only have an impact on subsequent miscarriage rate in patients with polycystic ovary syndrome who normally only can conceive after ovulation induction. Whether normalization of an abnormal BMI will improve the pregnancy prognosis in terms of miscarriage rate in these patients is still to be documented, but clearly, weight loss will decrease the risk of gestational diabetes and other late pregnancy complications.

Lifestyle Factors

The most important lifestyle factors of importance for RM are consumption of coffee, alcohol, and tobacco in addition to the extent of leisure-time exercise during pregnancy. Drug abuse is rare in RM women but should be monitored. Whereas information about coffee consumption is trustworthy, information about alcohol and tobacco use will probably be underestimated. In my clinic we tell patients that daily consumption of four or more cups of coffee (and tea and cola with an equivalent caffeine content) during pregnancy should be avoided since several studies have reported that this increases the risk of miscarriage in the general population.

Any use of alcohol at least in the first half of pregnancy should be strongly discouraged since just one to two drinks a week in the first trimester have been shown to double the miscarriage risk and there is also an increased risk of fetal alcohol syndrome.

Whereas there is no good proof that tobacco use increases the risk of early miscarriage, the patients should try to reduce smoking, primarily to diminish the risk of late pregnancy complications such as intrauterine growth retardation, preterm birth, and placental abruption – conditions strongly associated with both RM and smoking.

Information should be obtained about leisure-time exercise since recent research suggests that some kinds of high-impact exercise, defined as exercise more than 75 min a week, may increase miscarriage risk <14th week significantly with relative risks of 3.6–4.2 in pregnant women from the general population. Therefore, patients should be interviewed specifically about what kind of exercise they perform and for how many hours a week. If it is estimated that the patient practises too much "dangerous" exercise, she should be encouraged to reduce its intensity and duration.

Social Class

Low social class and low educational level are risk factors for perinatal complications such as preterm birth, which can only partly be explained by a more unhealthy lifestyle (high BMI, smoking, drinking) among low social class women. In my clinic, we ask the couples about their occupation and this information will in most instances provide a rough estimate of their social status. Whereas the social factors cannot be changed by interventions at the RM clinic, extra surveillance in the third trimester should be provided for some of these patients due to the higher risk of late pregnancy complications.

Occupational Factors

Patients should be interviewed in details about their working situation. Is their working situation very stressful? Are they standing many hours a day or are they lifting heavy burdens? Do they have changing working times including night work? Are they working with hazardous chemicals or radiation? Although the documentation that improvement of working conditions indeed improves perinatal outcome is poor, RM patients with risky work conditions should be encouraged to change the conditions and support be provided to implement the changes (letters to the employers, etc.). Patients with night work may be encouraged to only work by day time in the next pregnancy, diminish working load, or get pregnancy leave.

Partner

Patients with RM are almost always married or live in an established partnership. In my clinic, the husband is asked whether he has fathered pregnancies in previous relationships and about the outcome of these pregnancies. In addition, he is asked about health status with particular focus on congenital or testicular disorders and intake of medicine.

An increasing number of our RM couples are immigrants from the Middle East, with tradition for inter-cousin marriages. Therefore, it is important to obtain information about whether the couples are related. There may be an increased risk of miscarriage in first-cousin marriages and definitely an increased risk of malformations and autosomal recessive diseases in the offspring. This may be an indication for closer-than-normal ultrasonic fetal monitoring during pregnancy. If a first-cousin couple with RM continues to miscarry in spite of other treatments, the possibility of offering insemination with donor sperm should be mentioned to the couple, but due to culture and religion, this offer will rarely be accepted.

> ✋ CAUTION
>
> Most published studies put little emphasis on lifestyle and occupational factors, although these may affect pregnancy outcome more than factors found by blood tests.
>
> Too much emphasis should not be put on the importance of a moderately increased BMI since its impact on miscarriage risk in RM is unclear and the effect of weight loss on miscarriage risk is undocumented.
>
> Many patients with RM seek an explanation for their miscarriages in some self-inflicted factor, for example, intake of a specific food ingredient, a stressful event, a jump, or a heavy lift. Such self-guilt can be enhanced if the importance of lifestyle factors for RM is over-exaggerated when talking with the patients.

Reproductive history

Clinical Appearance of Pregnancy Losses

In my clinic, considerable time is spent to get valid information about the patients' reproductive history, especially about the gestational ages at the time of previous fetal demise and the ultrasonographic and hormonal measurements undertaken in each pregnancy. This information is obtained from questionnaires sent to the patients before the first consultation in order to give them time to collect relevant data from hospital records and other documents and to recall events.

At the first consultation, every effort is done to integrate information from written records and the patients' own information in order to answer four main questions relating to each pregnancy: (i) was it confirmed by a urinary pregnancy test or serum-hCG measurement? (ii) were there signs of intrauterine pregnancy by ultrasound (intrauterine gestational sac, yolk sac, or embryonal echo with or without fetal heart action)? (iii) were chorionic villi detected by histology after uterine curettage? and (iv) at which gestational age had the fetal demise probably happened?

Other information relating to previous pregnancies is also thoroughly collected: mode of conception, results from karyotyping of miscarriages, identity of the partner for each pregnancy, and perinatal data relating to pregnancies progressing to the second/third trimester. Any treatment attempts in each pregnancy are also registered.

Our efforts to register detailed data from previous pregnancies are primary due to the fact that the number of previous pregnancy losses is the strongest prognostic factor for further miscarriage/live birth after RM. It is thus important to confirm that the patients had really had pregnancy losses by documenting a positive urine or serum-hCG measurement and not merely irregular cycles. It is also important to know whether a pregnancy has been documented by ultrasound or histology and not only by hCG detection since biochemical pregnancies (also called pregnancies of unknown location = PULs) may influence the prognosis after RM differently from clinical miscarriages. Some gynecologists and specialist societies such as the American Society of Reproductive Medicine do not recognize the importance of PULs in the RM diagnosis. However, my group has documented that PULs in the reproductive history indeed matter – in a multivariate analysis of variables of importance for subsequent pregnancy outcome in 499 RM patients, each PUL reduced the prognosis for subsequent live birth significantly and almost to the same degree as each clinical miscarriage.

We also found that primary RM patients with a history of exclusively PULs exhibit a very high (16%) frequency of clinical tubal pregnancy at some time point in their reproductive history. This may indicate that the pregnancy losses in many of these patients may be spontaneously resorbed ectopic pregnancies due to tubal damage rather than intrauterine losses. We suspect that these patients have a subtotal tubal damage and as a consequence, we offer them IVF treatment in the next pregnancy – providing them with a good chance for live birth (see Chapters 8 and 17).

> ### ✋ CAUTION
>
> Some patients exaggerate the number of pregnancy losses in order to qualify for being referred to a dedicated RM clinic and qualify for active treatment at the clinic. These patients can be identified by doing an extensive collection of information from files from hospitals and general practitioners.

Gestational Age of Pregnancy Losses

Information about time of fetal demise, not to confound with the time of discovery of fetal death, is important, especially when we are dealing with pregnancy losses in the early second trimester (13th–18th week gestation). It has been reported in several studies that when fetal death is documented to have happened after 13th week, it is associated with a much higher risk of new second trimester miscarriage or extreme early birth compared with an early miscarriage (see Chapter 5). Some miscarriages detected by ultrasound in the second trimester have, evaluated from the size of the dead fetus, probably happened in the first trimester. Since the impact of a "real" second trimester loss on the risk of new late loss or preterm birth seems to be much greater than the impact of a first trimester loss, in my clinic much efforts are done to collect relevant information in order to distinguish between "real" and "false" second trimester losses in the history.

> ### ✭ TIPS AND TRICKS
>
> Questionnaires requesting information about time and place for previous pregnancy losses and about investigations undertaken in each pregnancy should be mailed to new patients 3 weeks prior to initial consultation.

Perinatal Data

Information about outcome of previous births or stillbirths is important to obtain. Our studies have shown that in patients with secondary RM, the birth of a boy compared with a girl prior to RM decreases the prognosis for live birth in the first pregnancy after referral by 22% corresponding to an OR for birth of 0.37 (95% CI 0.2–0.7). If the firstborn boy was born preterm or had birth weight <2500 g, the prognosis seems to be reduced even more.

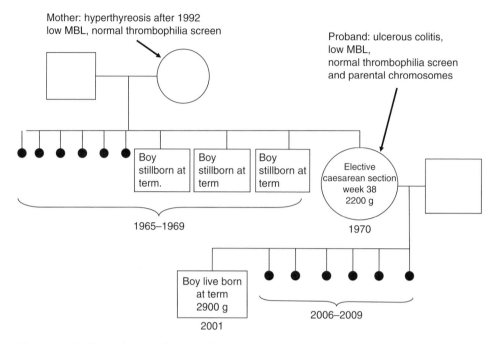

Figure 1.1 Pedigree showing the reproductive histories of a woman (proband) with secondary recurrent miscarriage after the birth of a slightly growth-retarded boy and her mother. Information about autoimmune diseases and screening for risk factors for recurrent miscarriage are also given. MBL, mannose-binding lectin.

The patient database at my clinic indicates that women with secondary RM significantly more often than expected had given birth to a firstborn child with some congenital disorder or malformation. In these cases, many efforts are done to achieve information about the exact diagnosis of the child and together with experts in genetics and ultrasound to make a plan for surveillance in the next pregnancy, including prenatal screening and, if possible, offer treatment with IVF combined with preimplantation genetic diagnosis (see Chapter 6).

Information about perinatal complications when the patients themselves were born can provide information about the prognosis for birth since women being born with a low own birth weight (<2900 g) will have a high risk of experiencing multiple (≥5) miscarriages in their later reproductive life (Figure 1.1).

> ⚙ **SCIENCE REVISITED**
>
> In the majority of published studies in RM, little emphasis is put on getting a comprehensive reproductive history with documentation of pregnancy losses being biochemical, early clinical miscarriages, or "real" second trimester miscarriages.
>
> Detailed information about the time of fetal demise in previous pregnancy losses and perinatal outcome in previous ongoing pregnancies is important for assessing the risk of new miscarriage and late pregnancy complications.

Disease history

A thorough history of disease must be obtained. We focus in particular on autoimmune diseases, which are clearly overrepresented in RM women. The endocrine and metabolic changes associated with some autoimmune diseases such as type I diabetes and hypothyreosis may in theory directly interfere with trophoblast invasion and growth; alternatively, the increased inflammatory cytokine response and breakage of immunological tolerance characterizing autoimmune disease is predisposing to miscarriage and RM. Whatever autoimmune disease a patient has, its presence strengthens the belief that immunological disturbances are causing the miscarriages also in patients negative for the limited panel of autoantibodies investigated in most RM clinics. The patients should also be asked about previous thromboembolic episodes; presence of such will strengthen the suspicion that the patient has a thrombophilic disorder even though the routine screening for thrombophilic factors is normal.

Family history

Collecting a family history, especially from RM women, has high priority in my clinic. During a period of 20 years, we have asked our patients for information about the reproductive histories of siblings and mothers and we found that also in families of patients with normal karyotypes, sisters, brothers' wives and mothers all displayed miscarriage rates that were almost doubled compared with the background population. In addition, we found that first-degree relatives had an increased prevalence of a series of autoimmune diseases. A high frequency of miscarriages, perinatal complications, and autoimmune disease among first-degree relatives may suggest that the patient origins from a family carrying genes for poor trophoblast development and genes predisposing to breakage of immunological tolerance and proinflammatory responses (Figure 1.1). Carriage of such genetic factors is probably associated with a diminished prognosis for live birth. An accumulation of miscarriage and autoimmune disease among the first-degree relatives should alert the general practitioner or nonspecialized gynecologist and lead to referral to a specialized RM clinic already after two or three miscarriages. A burdened family history should lead the physicians of the RM clinic to monitor the patients more closely during early and late pregnancy since the risk of miscarriage and perinatal complications in the patients' next pregnancy may be increased. A family history of early onset autoimmune or thromboembolic disease should alert the physician in the RM clinic about a possible immunological or thrombophilic etiology in spite of normal routine blood screening and this may warrant extended blood testing.

Information about repeated miscarriages among first-degree siblings or their mothers increases the chance that the patients carry a balanced translocation and based on this finding it has been proposed only to investigate karyotypes in younger RM patients with a family history of repeated miscarriages to save costs (see Chapter 2).

However, it must be emphasized that no study has so far attempted to quantify the impact of a family history of miscarriage, perinatal complications, or early onset autoimmune and thromboembolic disease for the risk of new miscarriage in patients with RM. When such a study has been undertaken, it will hopefully be possible to include family information in a more exact way when estimating the prognosis in patients with RM.

> **PEARLS TO TAKE HOME**
>
> A family history of repeated miscarriages or autoimmune or early onset thromboembolic disease should alert the physician of a diminished spontaneous prognosis, which should lead to referral to a dedicated RM clinic already after few (2–3) miscarriages.

Conclusions

As reviewed earlier, it is rewarding to spend efforts and time to get a comprehensive history from the patients. I think that a thorough reproductive history with detailed knowledge about whether the pregnancy loses had been PULs or clinical miscarriages, whether miscarriages had been before or after gestational week 13, and whether there had been perinatal complications associated with previous births is paramount for estimating the prognosis as exact as possible and thus will help in the decision taking regarding whether to treat or not. A reliable estimate of the number of previous pregnancy losses and their gestational ages is also important for assessing the risk of perinatal complications in subsequent ongoing pregnancies, which will influence the level of monitoring that should be offered in late pregnancy. Sometimes the reproductive history per se can be decisive for offering the patients IVF treatment or other kinds of assisted reproduction.

Clearly, if risk factors for miscarriages in the patients' lifestyle or occupation are identified, this should result in improvement of lifestyle and working conditions.

Information about autoimmune or thromboembolic disease among the patients themselves or their first-degree family members can often raise suspicion about a possible immunological or thrombophilic etiology of miscarriages in spite of normal routine blood screening, and this may lead to extended biochemical testing.

Figure 1.1 illustrates the value of obtaining a thorough disease and reproductive history concerning a RM patient and her first-degree family members. The patient was referred to our clinic after having experienced six early miscarriages after the birth of a growth-retarded boy. It was planned to offer her treatment with intravenous immunoglobulin (IvIg) in her next pregnancy but unfortunately 3 years after referral, she had not yet managed to conceive in spite of assisted reproductive technology (ART), probably due to advanced age (now 42 years). Her history with own low-birth weight, the birth of a growth-retarded boy in the first pregnancy, symptoms of autoimmune disease (ulcerous colitis), and her mother's history of several unexplained still-births (of growth-retarded boys), RM and autoimmune disease (hyperthyreosis) suggest that the family carries genetic variants that predispose both to autoimmunity and impaired trophoblast growth or function and points to a poor prognosis. We found that both the patient and her mother had very low plasma levels of mannose-binding lectin (MBL), which is determined by genetic polymorphisms on chromosome 10. Low MBL levels predispose to RM with reduced prognosis, late fetal death, and low-birth weight. The clinical information about the patient and her family was not very useful at the time when the patient was finally referred to our clinic because at that time she had become candidate for our most extensive therapy (IvIg), exclusively due to the high number of miscarriages. However, she did not get the chance to benefit from this treatment due to advanced age. If the information regarding the patient and her mother had been collected and taken seriously already when she had suffered her third miscarriage, she would have been referred at a time when she was still able to conceive and benefit from the possible effect of IvIg treatment (see Chapter 6).

Overall, a valid and detailed information about all the relevant factors that can be achieved from talking with the patients and reading their hospital records will, in conjunction with results from blood tests and investigations of uterine anatomy, provide the best basis for assessing the patients' prognosis, in terms of chance of life birth and risk of perinatal complications, and will help taking the decision about when and how to treat.

PATIENT ADVICE

If a risk factor for RM is identified in a patient, it is important to tell her that this is probably not the full explanation for the disorder but a piece in the jig jaw puzzle and eliminating or treating this factor is no guaranty for pregnancy success.

Bibliography

Christiansen, O.B., Steffensen, R., Nielsen, H.S. and Varming, K. (2008) Multifactorial etiology of recurrent miscarriage and its scientific and clinical implications. *Gynecologic Obstetric Investigation*, **66**, 257–267.

Edlow, A.G., Srinivas, S.K. and Elovitz, M.A. (2007) Second trimester loss and subsequent pregnancy outcomes: what is the real risk? *American Journal of Obstetrics Gynecology*, **197**, 581e1–581e6.

Kolte, A.M., Nielsen, H.S., Moltke, I. *et al.* (2011) A genome-wide scan in affected sibling pairs with idiopathic recurrent miscarriage suggests genetic link. *Molecular Human Reproduction*, **17**, 379–385.

Nielsen, H.S., Andersen, A.M., Kolte, A.M. *et al.* (2008) A first born boy is suggestive of a strong prognostic factor in secondary recurrent miscarriage – a confirmatory study. *Fertility and Sterility*, **89**, 907–911.

Which Investigations Are Relevant?

Paulien G. de Jong,[1] Emmy van den Boogaard,[2] Claudia R. Kowalik,[3]
Rosa Vissenberg,[2] Saskia Middeldorp[1] and Mariëtte Goddijn[2]

[1] Department of Vascular Medicine, Academic Medical Center, Amsterdam,
The Netherlands
[2] Center for Reproductive Medicine, Department of Obstetrics and Gynecology,
Academic Medical Center, Amsterdam, The Netherlands
[3] Department of Obstetrics and Gynecology, Academic Medical Center,
Amsterdam, The Netherlands

Introduction

Potential risk factors for a subsequent miscarriage can be identified in women with preceding recurrent miscarriage (RM). The strength of the association with RM is not clear for all risk factors. The question thus remains which diagnostic tests should be used in daily clinical practice. Ideally, diagnostic tests should only be carried out if the test can either give insight in the prognosis of the individual patient or if the established cause can be treated effectively.

In clinical practice, the decision to perform diagnostic investigations follows upon a detailed history with regard to the prior miscarriages and a further medical, obstetric, lifestyle, and family history.

Women with RM are often in great despair, and it is not uncommon that diagnostic investigations are being performed and treatments are being described despite a lack of evidence. It has been shown that too many diagnostic investigations and unproven treatments are performed in women with RM since doctors find it difficult to resist insistent women.

New medical tests should be thoroughly evaluated before they are introduced in routine clinical practice, this way avoiding erroneous diagnoses or alternatively, the initiation of unproven potentially harmful therapy. In addition, increasing costs of healthcare have been calling for the elimination of ineffective medical testing.

Presently, many diagnostic interventions for women or couples with RM are controversial because there is no information available with regard to prognosis and lack of evidence of potential treatment options in case of positive test results. There is a high need for prospective cohort studies for prognostic purposes and randomized, adequately powered trials to test the beneficial effects and absence of harmful effects of treatment interventions. Only after elucidating the prognosis for individual women and/or establishing a beneficial safe treatment effect, diagnostic investigations should be performed on a routine basis in clinical practice.

Chapter 2 of this book deals with the diagnostic investigations testing for thrombophilia, chromosome abnormalities, uterine abnormalities, and thyroid autoimmunity in women with RM.

EVIDENCE AT A GLANCE

- ESHRE guideline "recurrent miscarriage," 2006
- RCOG guideline "recurrent miscarriage, investigation and treatment of couples," 2011
- ACCP guideline "VTE, Thrombophilia, Antithrombotic Therapy, and Pregnancy" 2012

Thrombophilia tests

The term thrombophilia is used to describe a disorder associated with an increased tendency to venous thromboembolism (VTE). It can be acquired, as in women with malignant disease or antiphospholipid syndrome, as well as inherited. Traditionally, possible features are a family history of thrombosis, thrombosis at an unusual location or thrombosis at young age, but a large proportion of carriers of thrombophilic defects remains asymptomatic throughout life. In addition to these features, thrombophilia is also associated with an increased risk of both sporadic miscarriage and RM. Severe preeclampsia is also associated with thrombophilia; for other adverse pregnancy outcomes, including placental abruption and intrauterine growth restriction, the presence of an association is controversial.

Tests

The **antiphospholipid syndrome** is diagnosed in women if they test positive for lupus anticoagulant (nonspecific inhibitor), have moderate or high titre IgG or IgM anticardiolipin antibodies (>40 GPL or MPL or >99th percentile) or moderate or high titre IgG or IgM β2glycoprotein I antibodies (>99th percentile) on two occasions at least 12 weeks apart and suffer from at least one clinical criteria such as unexplained fetal death (later than 10 weeks of gestation), three or more unexplained consecutive miscarriages (before 10 weeks of gestation), or one or more premature births of a morphologically normal neonate before the thirty-fourth week of gestation because of eclampsia, severe preeclampsia, or placental insufficiency.

These criteria for diagnosis were decided at a consensus conference in Sydney in 2006 but as of yet, still more evidence-based data are needed to sharpen the criteria.

Inherited thrombophilias are diagnosed by laboratory testing if a factor V Leiden mutation or prothrombin gene mutation (G20210A) is present or if a deficiency of antithrombin, protein C, or protein S is present on two separate occasions and measured outside of pregnancy, combined oral contraceptive use, or significant liver disease.

> **✋ CAUTION**
>
> Antiphospholipid syndrome and inherited thrombophilia are associated with RM. Guidelines do not advise to test for all forms of thrombophilia, since a positive test result will not always alter clinical management.
>
> Antiphospholipid syndrome **is diagnosed** if tested positive, one two occasions at least 12 weeks apart, for:
>
> - lupus anticoagulant *or*
> - moderate or high titre IgG or IgM anticardiolipin antibodies (>40 GPL or MPL or >99th percentile) *or*
> - moderate or high titre IgG or IgM β2glycoprotein I antibodies (>99th percentile) on two occasions at least 12 weeks apart
> - *and* RM (three or more losses <10 weeks' gestation and or one or more losses >10 weeks' gestation)

Coagulation Cascade, Regulatory Mechanisms

Inherited thrombophilia can be explained by decreased levels of anticoagulant proteins or altered functions of coagulation factors due to mutations. The effects of the currently known inherited thrombophilic defects on fibrin formation are explained in Figure 2.1. The process of coagulation is activated and regulated in several ways, in which thrombin (factor IIa) plays a key role. It converts fibrinogen to fibrin; the main component of a hemostatic plug. Second, it activates coagulation factors V, VIII, XI, leading to increased thrombin formation, and factor XIII, which crosslinks fibrin strands. Coagulation is physiologically regulated by protein C and protein S. Protein C is activated to activated Protein C (APC) by thrombin in the presence of thrombomodulin. APC inactivates factors Va and VIIIa, and protein S serves as a cofactor in this process, indirectly decreasing thrombin formation. A third natural anticoagulant is antithrombin; it inhibits thrombin directly, but can also inactivate factors Xa, IXa, VIIa and plasmin, thereby indirectly inhibiting thrombin formation.

Inherited Thrombophilia

Two forms of inherited thrombophilia are the gain of functional mutations called factor V Leiden and prothrombin gene mutation (G20210A). Factor V Leiden results from a substitution of adenine for guanine at the 1691 position of the factor V gene. This leads to the substitution of glutamine for arginine at position 506 in the factor V polypeptide. As a consequence, factor Va is resistant to degradation by APC, which results in less downregulation of thrombin, compared to normal factor Va.

The prothrombin gene mutation results from a mutation in the promotor region of the prothrombin gene (G20210A), which leads to slightly elevated prothrombin levels, which is associated with an increased risk of thromboembolism.

Deficiencies of the natural anticoagulants antithrombin, protein C and protein S lead to increased thrombin generation and are relatively rare forms of inherited thrombophilia.

Prevalence of Inherited Thrombophilia

Altogether, the different forms of inherited thrombophilia are not rare, but the frequency varies considerably within healthy populations. Heterozygosity for factor V Leiden is

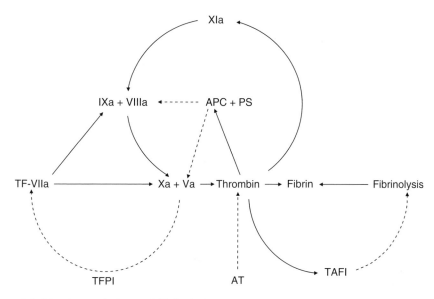

Figure 2.1 Blood coagulation and fibrinolysis.

Simplified scheme of coagulation and fibrinolysis. Coagulation is initiated by a tissue factor (TF)–factor VIIa complex that can activate factor IX or factor X, leading to formation of the key enzyme thrombin (factor IIa). Tissue factor-dependent coagulation is rapidly inhibited by tissue factor pathway inhibitor (TFPI). Coagulation is maintained through the activation of factor XI by thrombin. Through the intrinsic tenase complex (factors IXa and VIIIa) and the prothrombinase complex (factors Xa and Va), the additional thrombin required to downregulate fibrinolysis is generated by the activation of thrombin-activatable fibrinolysis inhibitor (TAFI). The coagulation system is regulated by the protein C pathway. Thrombin activates protein C in the presence of thrombomodulin. Together with protein S (PS), activated protein C (APC) is capable of inactivating factors Va and VIIIa, which results in a downregulation of thrombin generation and consequently in an upregulation of the fibrinolytic system. The activity of thrombin is controlled by the inhibitor antithrombin (AT). The solid arrows indicate activation and the broken arrows inhibition.

the most prevalent inherited thrombophilic defect, occurring in 5% of Caucasians; however, it is rare in Asians and Africans. The mutation in the prothrombin gene is present in approximately 2–3% of Caucasians, but is also less common in Asians and Africans. Homozygosity for these two mutations is rare, with a prevalence of 0.02% for factor V Leiden and 0.014% for prothrombin gene mutation (G20210A). Deficiencies of Protein C, Protein S, and antithrombin are much rarer than factor V Leiden or prothrombin gene mutation (G20210A); their combined prevalence is approximately 1%.

Pathophysiological Mechanisms Leading to Pregnancy Loss

Physiologically, pregnancy is associated with changes in hemostasis, resulting in a hypercoagulable state. In theory, thrombophilia intensifies these changes in hemostasis during pregnancy. The association between thrombophilia and RM as well as other pregnancy complications can therefore be explained by the concept of thrombosis of the (micro) vasculature of the placenta. This hypothesis is reinforced by the fact that placental infarction is a common finding in women with placenta-mediated pregnancy complications and thrombophilia.

However, it is unlikely that this is the sole mechanism of thrombophilia in miscarriage. Because placental development has not yet taken place very early in pregnancy and early miscarriage is also associated with thrombophilia, other pathophysiological mechanisms may also play a part.

A suggested mechanism by which antiphospholipid syndrome induces injury to the developing fetal–placental unit is by activation of complement. In animal models, binding of antiphospholipid antibodies to trophoblast can activate complement factors C3 and C5, leading to recruitment and stimulation of inflammatory cells and injury to the fetus and placenta. Furthermore, in in vitro studies on human placental tissue, it was demonstrated that antiphospholipid antibodies can inhibit primary extravillous trophoblast differentiation, and subsequent placentation. Finally, it is observed that heparin as well as aspirin regulates trophoblast apoptosis in vitro.

Similar experimental models for *inherited* thrombophilia have not been studied, but experiments on thrombomodulin-deficient mice have shown that the thrombomodulin–protein C pathway is essential for the maintenance of pregnancy; activated coagulation factors induce cell death and growth inhibition of placental trophoblast cells by formation of fibrin degradation products, inducing death of giant trophoblast cells, as well as by engaging protease-activated receptors PAR-2 and PAR-4. These findings suggest that the thrombomodulin–protein C system may protect placental integrity, and consequently, that a lack of protein C can be a partial explanation of pregnancy loss.

Strength of the Association

The effect of thrombophilic defects on pregnancy outcome seems to vary for different forms of thrombophilia and during the course of pregnancy (see Table 2.1).

The association between pregnancy complications, such as premature birth or eclampsia and the presence of antiphospholipid antibodies is less clear than for RM.

One study reported an association between increased risk of RM throughout the first trimester and prothrombin gene mutation G20210A, whereas factor V Leiden was associated with RM after the start of placentation (10–14 weeks gestation), but not with embryonic loss. A meta-analysis showed that RM with only first trimester miscarriages is associated with factor V Leiden and prothrombin G20210A mutation. Late pregnancy loss was associated with factor V Leiden (pregnancy loss >19 weeks gestational age), prothrombin G20210A mutation (loss >20 weeks), and protein S deficiency (loss >22 weeks). The association between factor V Leiden and late RM was stronger than for early RM (<13 weeks). Results of another systematic review showed that women with unexplained stillbirth were more often heterozygous for factor V Leiden, or had protein S deficiency more often than controls.

Anticoagulant Therapy; Evidence and Drawbacks

Recently performed randomized controlled trials (RCTs) investigated the effect of anticoagulant therapy on subsequent live birth in women with a history of *unexplained* RM. It was found that neither aspirin combined with low molecular weight heparin (LMWH) nor aspirin alone improved the chance of a live birth in women with a history of unexplained RM.

Table 2.1 Association Between Pregnancy Complications and Thrombophilia (4)

Type of Thrombophilia	Miscarriage (first or second trimester) OR (95% CI)	Recurrent First Trimester Miscarriage OR (95% CI)	Nonrecurrent Second Trimester Miscarriage OR (95% CI)	Stillbirth (third trimester loss) OR (95% CI)
Factor V Leiden (homozygous)	2.7 (1.3–5.6)	*	*	2.0 (0.4–9.7)
Factor V Leiden (heterozygous)	1.7 (1.1–2.6)	1.9* (1.0–3.6)	4.1* (1.9–8.8)	2.1 (1.1–3.9)
Prothrombin gene mutation (heterozygous)	2.5 (1.2–5.0)	2.7 (1.4–5.3)	8.6 (2.2–34.0)	2.7 (1.3–5.5)
Antithrombin deficiency	0.9 (0.2–4.5)	NA	NA	7.6 (0.3–196.4)
Protein C deficiency	2.3 (0.2–26.4)	NA	NA	3.1 (0.2–38.5)
Protein S deficiency	3.6 (0.4–35.7)	NA	NA	20.1 (3.7–109.2)
Anticardiolipin antibodies	3.4 (1.3–8.7)	5.1 (1.8–14.0)	NA	3.3 (1.6–6.7)
Lupus anticoagulants (Nonspecific inhibitor)	3.0 (1.0–8.6)	NA	14.3 (4.7–43.2)	2.4 (0.8–7.0)

*Homozygous and heterozygous carriers were grouped together; it is not possible to extract data for zygosity
NA, not available.
Note: data are derived from a systematic review; terminology of pregnancy loss at various gestational ages may vary among included studies. de Jong PG, Goddijn M, Middeldorp S. Testing for inherited thrombophilia in recurrent miscarriage. *Seminars in Reproductive Medicine* 2011; 29: 540–547.

For women with *antiphospholipid syndrome* based on the clinical criteria of a single late pregnancy loss, preeclampsia or fetal growth restriction, there is no evidence of an effect of anticoagulants (both heparin/aspirin). Nevertheless, for women with three or more miscarriages and antiphospholipid antibodies, evidence suggests that anticoagulants increase the chance of live birth in a subsequent pregnancy. A trend toward higher live birth rates was observed in women treated with LMWH in addition to aspirin in two small studies. Combined data from five trials testing the efficacy of heparin (either unfractionated heparin (UFH) or LMWH) with aspirin compared to aspirin alone showed a significant higher live birth rate in the heparin and aspirin group. As the effectiveness of LMWH in addition to aspirin is suggested to be at least equivalent to UFH in addition to aspirin, current guidelines recommend antepartum UFH or LMWH with aspirin over no treatment antepartum for women with antiphospholipid syndrome and three or more miscarriages.

None of the performed studies were sufficiently powered to demonstrate an effect of pharmacological therapy in the subgroup of women with *inherited thrombophilia*.

There is a need for randomized, adequately powered placebo-controlled trials on the use of anticoagulants in women with RM and inherited thrombophilia. Until beneficial effects of anticoagulants are demonstrated in such trials, pharmacological intervention in women with RM and inherited thrombophilia is not justified.

Fortunately, the risks of hemorrhage (including postpartum hemorrhage), heparin-induced thrombocytopenia (HIT), and heparin-induced osteopenia, which comprise the main potential adverse effects of heparins, appears to be small. Nevertheless, LMWH needs to be injected and administration often causes pain and bruising at injection sites. It is important to keep in mind that though anticoagulant therapy can be beneficial in specific cases, it is potentially harmful.

⚘ SCIENCE REVISITED

Current guidelines:

- Recommend prophylactic LMWH combined with low-dose aspirin (75–100 mg/day) for women who fulfill the laboratory criteria for antiphospholipid syndrome and meet the clinical criteria based on a history of three or more miscarriages
- Suggest not to use antithrombotic prophylaxis in women with inherited thrombophilia and a history of pregnancy complications

---

Screening for thrombophilia in women with recurrent miscarriage

Recognizing the association between RM and thrombophilia and the possible benefits of anticoagulant therapy, the question is raised whether testing women with RM for thrombophilia should be performed routinely. Arguments in favor of testing include the knowledge of the possible cause of miscarrying. This provides an explanation for the patient and her partner, as well as for her physician. A second and more important argument supportive of testing for thrombophilia, is to identify the group of women who could benefit from anticoagulant therapy in a future pregnancy.

A complete inherited thrombophilia screen is costly. Moreover, the psychological impact and societal consequences for a person knowing that she is a carrier of a (genetic) thrombophilic defect are potential drawbacks of testing. Studies have shown that women report to be more worried with the knowledge of being a carrier of thrombophilia and have problems with getting insured.

As described, for women who suffered from RM and test positive for antiphospholipid antibodies, evidence suggests that anticoagulant therapy increases the chance of a live birth in a future pregnancy. Therefore, testing for antiphospholipid syndrome in these women is recommended.

For inherited thrombophilia however, this is not the case. As yet, evidence for the efficacy of anticoagulants in women with inherited thrombophilia and RM is lacking. Since treatment of these women is, at present, not justified, testing for inherited thrombophilia should not alter clinical management and, therefore, should not be carried out.

Conclusions

Antiphospholipid syndrome and inherited thrombophilias are associated with RM, but at present, the strength and pathophysiology of the association are not fully elucidated. In specific situations, the use of anticoagulants will provide a means of increasing the chance of a live birth in women with RM. However, as yet, this beneficial effect is only suggested in women with RM and antiphospholipid syndrome, and physicians should refrain from prescribing heparins to women for solely the indication of unexplained RM with or without *inherited* thrombophilia.

Since it still remains to be established whether subsequent therapy will improve clinical outcome, the knowledge of a woman's inherited thrombophilic status should not alter clinical management, and testing for inherited thrombophilia should not be performed on a routine base, but only in the context of scientific studies.

Parental and fetal karyotyping

Parental Chromosome Abnormalities

Phenotypically normal persons can be carrier of a structural chromosome abnormality. Such abnormalities can be subdivided into translocations, inversions, deletions and duplications, of which translocations and inversions have the ability to be inherited also in a balanced form. In the balanced form, the overall package of genetic material is maintained. This allows for the possibility to reproduce, and offspring may be normal, balanced, or unbalanced. An unbalanced structural chromosome abnormality often results in a miscarriage.

Parental Chromosome Abnormalities and Recurrent Miscarriage

RM is associated with carrier status in one of the partners, most frequently balanced chromosome translocations followed by chromosome inversions. One of the reasons to offer karyotyping is to identify an underlying reason for the miscarriages.

Other reasons might be to find an explanation for the recurrence of the miscarriages, prognostic reasons, for example to investigate the chances of delivering a healthy child and the risk of a future miscarriage, and furthermore to reduce anxiety and distress by excluding carrier status as a likely cause of the RMs.

Women appear to be more frequently carriers than men. The prevalence of carrier status for balanced chromosome abnormalities has been reported to increase from approximately 0.7% in the general population to 2.2% after one miscarriage, 4.8% after two miscarriages, and up to 5.2% after three miscarriages. Overall, the prevalence of structural chromosome abnormalities in couples with RMs is reported to be 3–5%, dependent on the definition of RMs that is used and the criteria of chromosome abnormalities included.

More recent evidence offers the possibility to identify couples with an increased risk (>2.2% and up to 10%) of chromosome abnormalities based on four independent risk factors: maternal age at the time of the second miscarriage, two versus three or more miscarriages, a history of RM in parents and a history of RM in brothers or sisters of either partner. A model based on these four factors was developed to calculate the probability of carrier status more accurately.

Testing

Postnatal karyotyping in both parents can be performed by blood tests. Postnatal karyotyping is a reliable test. Since it is a laborious and time-consuming procedure to detect translocations, costs are around 1400 euro for both partners.

Reproductive consequences of carrier status

It should be emphasized that the test result will have no medical consequences for the health of the carrier him- or herself. It is important when counseling men or women who are carriers of a balanced chromosome translocation, to stress the absence of medical consequences for the carriers themselves as couples not infrequently have the perception to carry a severe disease. The products of conception in carriers can have a normal karyotype, the same karyotype as the carrier parent, or an unbalanced karyotype. As described, the latter can lead to miscarriage, stillbirth, or the birth of a child with major congenital impairments.

At the time when the relationship between RM and carrier status was just recognized, couples were counseled about their increased risk of miscarriages and unbalanced offspring. However, risk for unbalanced offspring was mainly based on theoretical models and prevalence known from other groups of carriers. More recent studies show that the risk of unbalanced offspring in carrier couples appears to be rather low (0.7%). Among 550 pregnancies in 247 couples with RM who were carriers of a chromosome translocation, only two viable unbalanced chromosome abnormalities were detected at prenatal diagnosis (0.35%), followed by induced abortion and birth of two children with an unbalanced karyotype (0.35%). This is a small risk when compared to the general risk for Down's syndrome, especially in older women. In all women with RM, with both positive and negative carrier status, the risk of unbalanced progeny is not increased (0.02%) compared to women from the general population (0.07%). In couples with RM, the cumulative chance of a healthy live birth is the same for carrier couples as in noncarrier couples. The only difference is that carrier couples are more often confronted with more miscarriages prior to a live birth. This increased frequency of miscarriages could be regarded as a rescue mechanism, to prevent an implanted but abnormal pregnancy from further growth.

Carriers detected through a history of RM seem to form a different subgroup within all carriers and are facing other reproductive risks than carriers detected through a previous birth of a child with an unbalanced karyotype or the birth of an unbalanced offspring in the family. Viable unbalanced offspring is hardly ever detected through a history of RM. The subgroup with RM is mainly prone for miscarriages and counselling should therefore focus on this risk rather than on the risk of unbalanced offspring.

Apart from gynecologists, clinical geneticists could also inform carrier couples about their good reproductive chances, with an increased risk of miscarriages and an increased but still very low risk of unbalanced offspring.

Treatment or prevention

Still, the risk of viable unbalanced offspring resulting from carrier status has always been the most important reason to offer parental chromosome testing. Regarding the low prevalence of unbalanced offspring, testing would be more justified if accurate treatment or accurate prevention would be available. Balanced chromosome abnormalities themselves cannot be treated of course. Carrier couples are generally offered prenatal diagnostics (PND) through amniocentesis or chorionic villus sampling to identify an unbalanced fetal karyotype. A complicating factor is that such an amniocentesis or chorionic villus sampling may lead to a procedure-related risk, 0.5–1% of a pregnancy loss. This is regarded as a highly unwanted risk for couples that were already confronted with miscarriages in the past, and more or less equals the risk of an unbalanced viable pregnancy. A cohort study has shown that many carrier couples refrain from PND in their next pregnancy.

It has been suggested to offer preimplantation genetic diagnostics (PGD) to carrier couples. This procedure includes an ICSI procedure with testing of the embryo for the unbalanced structural abnormality prior to embryo transfer. The aim of PGD would be to decrease the incidence of unbalanced offspring and reduce the risk of miscarriages. However, although the theory sounds plausible, review of the data does not show such results of PGD in practice. In a recently published systematic review, no randomized controlled trials or nonrandomized comparative studies comparing the effects of PGD with natural conception were found. Data could only be derived from observational studies and case reports. It was concluded that there is insufficient data indicating that PGD improves the live birth rate in women with carrier couples with RM compared with natural conception. The expensive and stressful treatment of PGD has therefore no place in the treatment of carrier couples with RM. In case of concomitant subfertility leading to an IVF/ICSI treatment, the balance of outweighing benefits versus risks could be more in favor of a positive decision toward PGD. However, even in this situation, it should be kept in mind that existing data do not support the use of PGD because there is no convincing evidence that it improves live birth rates.

Fetal karyotype

In maximum half of all pregnancies that end up in a miscarriage, the fetal karyotype is abnormal. This mainly concerns numerical chromosome abnormalities. The incidence of abnormal fetal karyotype is about the same in sporadic as in RMs. With an increase of maternal age at the time of conception, the risk of offspring with chromosomal abnormalities such as Down's syndrome also increases. As a result, the risk of miscarriage is related to maternal age.

Testing the Fetal Karyotype

To karyotype fetal tissue samples after a miscarriage is not as easy as postnatal parental karyotyping, since the tissue to be studied is often not vital and it may suffer from culture failure. Costs for fetal karyotyping are around 700 euro. Studies on modern techniques like comparative genomic hybridization (array-CGH), fluorescence in situ hybridization (FISH), multiplex ligation-dependent probe amplification (MLPA), and Quantitative fluorescent polymerase chain reaction (QF-PCR) did not yet improve the success rate of fetal karyotyping.

Prognostic Value and Treatment

The value of knowing the result of the fetal karyotype is debatable. It does not predict anything for the next pregnancy. It does also not exclude other underlying risks. For example, an abnormal fetal karyotype does not exclude antiphospholipid syndrome in the mother. The only value is to (partly) explain the parents the reason for the specific miscarriage in case of an abnormal fetal karyotype. There are studies suggesting that the risk of miscarriage is lower in the next pregnancy after a miscarriage with an abnormal fetal karyotype compared with a pregnancy after a miscarriage with a normal karyotype, but these studies need a proper evaluation by meta-analysis or IPD, taking into account maternal underlying factors.

☝ CAUTION

Fetal and parental karyotyping in couples with RM are expensive tests that do not reduce the incidence of unbalanced offspring. In women with RM, without other adverse outcomes like children born with multiple congenital handicaps, parental karyotyping can be withheld. If a couple has other risk factors for chromosome abnormalities – for example unbalanced offspring in the family, these could be an indication for parental chromosome testing.

⚙ SCIENCE REVISITED

Current guidelines:

- Advise to refrain from parental karyotyping in RM *only* (RCOG 2011) or test only in case of increased risk based on obstetric and family history (ESHRE 2006).
- Advise to refrain from standard fetal karyotyping (ESHRE 2006).
- The expensive and stressful treatment of PGD has no place in the treatment of carrier couples with RM.

PATIENT ADVICE

- Family history of children born with chromosome abnormalities is important for identifying risk factors. This could be an indication for parental karyotyping
- Fetal karyotyping is not indicated in women with RM

Conclusions

Couples with RM have an increased risk to be carrier of a chromosome abnormality. Carrier couples have an increased risk of another miscarriage. When compared to noncarriers with RM, the cumulative chance of healthy offspring is the same in both groups. The risk for unbalanced offspring in couples with RM is very low and equals the population risk prior to parental karyotyping and one can therefore refrain from routine parental karyotyping. Parental karyotyping should only be offered in case of other risk factors, for example the previous birth of a child with malformations or unbalanced offspring in the family.

Testing for fetal karyotype is not naturally followed by therapeutic implications and should only be performed within the setting of clinical research. Treatment with PGD does not increase reproductive chances in carrier couples.

Tests for diagnosing uterine anomalies

Congenital Uterine Anomalies

Congenital uterine anomalies are anomalies of the female reproductive system arising due to disturbances in formation, fusion and reabsorption of the Müllerian (paramesonephric) ducts. These Müllerian ducts are embryologic structures, which develop to form the fallopian tubes, the uterus, and the upper portion of the vagina in the female embryo. Disturbances in this complex embryologic development lead to various types of congenital uterine anomalies.

Failure of one of the Müllerian ducts to develop will result in a unicorn uterus or a uterus with a rudimentary horn. This rudimentary horn is sometimes lined with endometrium, but can develop without a cavity as well. It may communicate or not with the other half of the uterus.

When the Müllerian ducts fail to fuse, the uterus becomes *didelphic, bicornuate, or arcuate*. It depends on the degree of the fusion defect, which of these anomalies will arise. All of the anomalies due to fusion defects have a visible indentation on the external contour of the uterus.

The *septate uterus* results from a reabsorption defect of the midline septum. This anomaly has fused Müllerian ducts, but a division of the uterine cavity remains. The external contour of the uterus shows no abnormalities.

Since the congenital anomalies are a miscellaneous group of anomalies, various classification systems have been developed to order them. There is no universal agreement on which classification system should be used to classify them.

✋ CAUTION

Uterine anomalies are associated with adverse pregnancy outcome, like miscarriage and preterm birth. Testing will not alter treatment in women with RM yet, since there is insufficient evidence justifying the treatment of uterine anomalies to improve live birth rate.

Uterine Anomalies and Pregnancy Outcomes

All uterine anomalies have a negative effect on pregnancy outcomes.

The unicornuate and bicornuate uterus are associated with an increased risk of preterm birth and malpresentation at delivery. The arcuate uterus increases the risk of second trimester miscarriage and malpresentation at birth. The septate uterus is associated with subfertility, fetal malpresentation at delivery, an increased risk of first trimester miscarriage, and RM.

The septate uterus is the most common anomaly associated with one or more miscarriages, with a prevalence of 5.3% (95% CI 1.7–16.8), followed by the bicornuate uterus 2.1% (95% CI 1.4–3), both with prevalences being increased compared to women from the unselected population. The percentages may even be higher in women having experienced at least one miscarriage together with a history of subfertility. The prevalence of arcuate uteri of 2.9% (95% CI 0.9–9.6) is not increased after one or more miscarriages compared to women from the unselected population. A septate uterus is associated with the worst reproductive outcome of all uterine anomalies.

Diagnosis of uterine anomalies

Various diagnostic tests are available to diagnose an uterine anomaly, but not all tests are accurate and reliable. It is important to visualize the external and internal contour of the uterus when diagnosing a uterine anomaly. An anomaly cannot be accurately classified if information regarding the uterine fundus or cavity is lacking.

The gold standard for the diagnosis of a uterine anomaly is a laparoscopy or laparotomy combined with hysteroscopy. Other reliable tests are three-dimensional ultrasound, magnetic resonance imaging (MRI), and saline or gel infusion sonography (SIS/GIS).

Prognosis of pregnancy outcome

The prognosis of pregnancy outcome in the individual patient in whom a uterine anomaly has been diagnosed is difficult to establish. As described earlier, these women are at increased risk of another miscarriage. A septate uterus has the most detrimental effect, with increased risk of RM.

> ✋ **CAUTION**
>
> Congenital anomalies of the female reproductive tract are often associated with congenital anomalies of the urinary tract. If a uterine anomaly has been diagnosed, further investigations regarding the urinary tract should be performed.

Treatment of Uterine Anomalies

Surgical treatment of uterine anomalies is controversial. Research has most frequently focused on the surgical treatment of a septate uterus. This is due to the fact that the septate uterus is the most frequent anomaly associated with the highest risk on another miscarriage and most amenable to hysteroscopic surgery.

The underlying hypothesis of treatment of the septate uterus is that hysteroscopic resection of the septum (metroplasty) will restore normal anatomy and therefore uterine function. There is insufficient evidence to support this hypothesis however. The studies reported in literature are mostly retrospective studies using women with RM and a septate uterus as their own controls. However, this methodological set up is prone to bias. Women with a septate uterus and RM have a good chance of conceiving and a successful pregnancy without any intervention. When they serve within a cohort study as their own controls, this may affect the outcome, making it impossible to conclude if improvement in pregnancy outcome is due to the intervention or due to chance. RCTs are warranted to study whether surgical treatment of the septate uterus will improve live birth rate and is not harmful.

Conclusion

All uterine anomalies appear to have negative effects on reproductive outcome. Diagnostic tests are available to diagnose uterine anomalies, identifying women at risk for adverse pregnancy outcome, like another miscarriage or preterm birth.

Of all congenital uterine anomalies, a septate uterus appears to be associated with the highest risk of miscarrying again. Surgical treatment of the septate uterus is controversial, since there is insufficient evidence if surgical therapy will improve live birth rate and should be refrained from unless in the context of a randomized clinical trial. The knowledge of the presence of a septate uterus will not alter treatment in women with RM and a septate uterus. Therefore, routine testing for uterine anomalies in women with RM is not warranted but should be encouraged in the context of a research setting.

PATIENT ADVICE

- Uterine anomalies are common in women with RM
- For now it is unclear if surgical therapy will improve live birth rate. Routine testing for uterine anomalies is therefore not indicated in women with RM but only in the setting of scientific trials

---

Thyroid function tests

Thyroid Disorders

Different forms of thyroid disorders exist. Clinical hyperthyroidism and hypothyroidism are the best-known thyroid disorders. The diagnosis of clinical hyperthyroidism is based on a decreased thyroid stimulating hormone (TSH) with an increased free T4. The diagnosis of clinical hypothyroidism is based on high TSH concentrations and a decreased free T4. These women often present with symptoms. Clinical hyperthyroidism and hypothyroidism have proven to be associated with miscarriage, but not with RM.

Subclinical hypothyroidism, when there is a high TSH concentration, in combination with a normal free T4 level, is not associated with miscarriage or RM. The prevalence of these three thyroid disorders in women with RM is low, 1–2%.

In the last few years, research has focused on thyroid autoimmunity. Thyroid auto-immunity is defined as the presence of thyroid antibodies against thyroperoxidase (TPO antibodies) and/or thyroglobulin (Tg antibodies) in combination with a normal thyroid function, or euthyroid state. Women present without any symptoms, or symptoms are not easily recognized. TPO antibodies are normally present in about 90% of the women with a primary hypothyroidism or autoimmune thyroiditis, Hashimoto's disease. TPO is an enzyme expressed mainly in the thyroid that normally plays an important role in the production of thyroid hormones, thyroxine (T_4) or triiodo-thyronine (T_3). Thyroid autoimmunity has a prevalence of approximately 8–14% among women of fertile age. A higher prevalence has been described for women with RM, varying between 19 and 37%. TPO antibodies are far more frequently found than Tg antibodies. There is strong evidence of an association between thyroid autoimmunity and RM: a systematic review described an odds ratio of 2.5 (95% CI 1.6–3.9).

> **⚖ SCIENCE REVISITED**
>
> Thyroid autoimmunity is defined as the presence of thyroid antibodies against thyroperoxidase in combination with a normal thyroid function, or euthyroid state.
>   Several hypotheses exist on the causality between thyroid autoimmunity and RM:
>
> 1. The presence of autoantibodies reflects a generalized activation of the immune system.
> 2. Thyroid autoimmunity is associated with subfertility and more often found in women of higher age and therefore associated with RM.
> 3. Recurrent miscarriage is secondary to a subtle deficiency in thyroid hormone concentrations or a lower capacity of the thyroid to adequately adapt to the demands of pregnancy.

Diagnosis of Thyroid Disorders

Thyroid disorders can be diagnosed by the assessment of serum TSH, T4, or TPO antibody levels. Only one assessment is enough to diagnose a thyroid disorder. The test has a high sensitivity and specificity, ranging between 93% and 100%. Around 60% of women with thyroid autoimmunity have presence of TPO antibodies only, 5% have Tg antibodies only, and 35% have both TPO antibodies and Tg antibodies. If Tg antibodies are found, then in most cases, also TPO antibodies are present. For this reason, assessment of TPO antibodies is sufficient to diagnose thyroid autoimmunity. The diagnosis of thyroid disorders is complicated because different cutoff levels and different assays are being used. The available assay methods have a high sensitivity and specificity and are very similar. It is unclear which reference interval is normal for women of fertile age who wish to conceive or are pregnant. This is further complicated by the physiological change of the thyroid function during pregnancy. TSH and free T4 levels are lower in pregnant women, especially in the first trimester, and in the second and third trimester TSH levels are decreased. Besides, there are ethnic differences in thyroid function. For now, standardized or trimester-specific reference intervals are unavailable. Geographical differences in iodine intake can complicate standardization of reference intervals. For TPO antibodies, the most commonly used cutoff levels are 60 kU/l or 100 kU/l, but no consensus exist on the best cutoff level.

Thyroid Autoimmunity and Pregnancy Outcomes

Not much is known about pregnancy outcomes in women with RM and thyroid autoimmunity. For women with thyroid autoimmunity, it has been proven to be associated with subfertility, preterm birth, and maternal postpartum thyroid disease, but no studies have focused on pregnancy outcomes for women with RM and thyroid autoimmunity. There is no evidence whether there is a difference in live birth rates in the next pregnancy for women with RM and thyroid autoimmunity compared to women with RM without thyroid autoimmunity. Only one prospective cohort study is available on this topic describing 162 women with thyroid antibodies. This study showed no difference in live birth rates.

Treatment of Thyroid Autoimmunity

There is scarce evidence about treatment interventions for thyroid autoimmunity.

It seems that treatment with levothyroxine lowers the risk for miscarriage and preterm birth in women with thyroid autoimmunity, but this is only based on two small studies. Treatment with selenium is not effective in preventing postpartum thyroid disease, but the evidence is poor. It should be realized that no studies are available for a RM population. Live birth rate has never been studied as an outcome.

> ✋ **CAUTION**
>
> Although thyroid autoimmunity is associated with RM, guidelines do not advise standard testing for thyroid autoimmunity. The reason is insufficient evidence that treatment with levothyroxine improves live birth rates. Testing for thyroid autoimmunity is justified in a research setting.

Screening for Thyroid Autoimmunity

Different guidelines exist on RM. The European Society of Human Reproduction and Embryology (ESHRE) guideline "recurrent miscarriage" (2006) does not mention screening of thyroid disease in women with RM. The Royal College of Obstetricians and Gynaecologists (RCOG) guideline "The Investigation and Treatment of Couples with Recurrent First-trimester and Second-trimester Miscarriage" (2011) mentions thyroid autoimmunity but also that the evidence about this topic is poor, level 3. This guideline advises not to screen for thyroid auto-immunity. This is based on a single study, published in 1998, that has reported that women with RMs are no more likely than women without RM to have circulating thyroid antibodies. This is not in agreement with the results of the previous mentioned systematic review, published in 2011, where meta-analysis was performed on nine more recently published studies. A prospective study showed that the presence of thyroid antibodies in euthyroid women with a history of RM does not affect future pregnancy outcome, and strengthens the recommendation to refrain from routine screening for TPO antibodies.

Further Research on Thyroid Autoimmunity

It is clear that more research needs to be done on the clinical consequences of thyroid autoimmunity in women with RM. There in not enough information about live birth rate and pregnancy outcomes for this specific population. RCTs are highly warranted to study the effect of treatment interventions on pregnancy outcomes. When more evidence is available, guidelines can give an evidence-based advise whether to screen for thyroid autoimmunity, and if treatment and which treatment of thyroid autoimmunity is effective. This will improve patient care as well. For now, thyroid function tests are only justified in a research setting.

Conclusions

Thyroid autoimmunity is associated with RM. The evidence about obstetric outcomes and treatment interventions once thyroid autoimmunity is detected is poor. For this reason, it is still advised not to screen routinely for thyroid autoimmunity in women with RM. RCTs and cohort studies are needed to study potential safe treatment interventions and future pregnancy outcome.

> **PATIENT ADVICE**
> - Family history of thyroid disorders may be an important risk factor.
> - Routinely screening of thyroid disorders is not indicated since it is unclear if and which therapy will improve live birth rate in women with RM.
> - Screening of thyroid disorders is only advised in case of complaints likely to be caused by these disorders or in the setting of scientific trials.

Summary

Diagnostic tests should only be carried out if the test can either give insight in the prognosis of future pregnancy outcomes of the individual woman or if the established cause can be treated effectively. Presently, many diagnostic interventions are controversial because of lack of supplying prognostic information or lack of evidence of a beneficial treatment option. Only testing for antiphospholipid antibodies is recommended in daily clinical practice since a beneficial effect of anticoagulant treatment has been described (Table 2.2). Testing for inherited thrombophilia, uterus anomalies, and thyroid autoimmunity is recommended within the setting of clinical trials (Table 2.3).

Testing for parental chromosome abnormalities should be avoided since no more potentially viable children with an unbalanced chromosome abnormality are detected in women with RM compared to women from the general population. Testing for fetal chromosome abnormalities does not change clinical practice and should not be routinely performed (Table 2.4).

Table 2.2 Relevant Diagnostic Investigations in Women with Recurrent Miscarriage in Daily Clinical Practice

Tests	Testing For	Clinical Consequences in Case of Abnormal Test Result
Antiphospolipid antibodies • Lupus anticoagulants • Anticardiolipin antibodies (IgM and IgG) • ß2 glycoprotein I antibodies (IgG and IgM)	Antiphospholipid syndrome	Anticoagulant treatment in subsequent pregnancy in the presence of clinical criteria of three or more miscarriages

Table 2.3 Diagnostic Investigations only Relevant in Setting of Scientific Studies for Women with Recurrent Miscarriage

Tests	Testing For	Clinical Consequences
Thrombophilia screening • Factor V Leiden mutation • Prothrombin G20210A mutation • Antithrombin • Protein C • Protein S	Inherited thrombophilia	Participation in clinical trials for evaluating anticoagulant treatment
Screening for septate uterus • 3D US • Saline/gel infusion sonography • MRI	Septate uterus	Participating in clinical trials for evaluating the effect of hysteroscopic metroplasty (surgical resection of the uterine septum)
Thyroid autoimmunity screening • TPO antibodies	Thyroid autoimmunity	Participating in clinical trials for evaluating treatment with levothyroxine

Table 2.4 Irrelevant Diagnostic Investigations for Women with Recurrent Miscarriage in Daily Clinical Practice

Tests	Testing For	Clinical Consequences
Parental karyotyping (male/female partner)	Structural chromosome abnormalities	No more handicapped children born after screening RM population compared to general population
Fetal karyotyping	Structural and numerical chromosome abnormalities.	Identifying the cause of current miscarriage
Submicroscopic genetic fetal testing (array-CGH, FISH, MLPA, QF-PCR)	Submicroscopic genetic disorders	Identifying a potential cause of current miscarriage. These tests did not yet improve the detection rate of fetal karyotyping

Bibliography

Bates, S.M., Greer, I.A.,and Middeldorp, S. *et al.* (2012) VTE, thrombophilia, antithrombotic therapy and pregnancy: antithrombotic therapy and prevention of thrombosis, 9th ed: American College of Chest Physicians Evidence-Based Clinical Practice Guidelines. *Chest* 141(2_suppl): e691S-e736S.

de Jong, P.G., Goddijn, M. and Middeldorp, S. (2011) Testing for inherited thrombophilia in recurrent miscarriage. *Seminars in Reproductive Medicine*, **29**, 540–547.

Jauniaux, E., Farquharson, R.G., Christiansen, O.B. and Exalto, N. (2006) European Society of Human Reproduction and Embryology (ESHRE). Evidence-based guidelines for the investigation and medical treatment of recurrent miscarriage. *Human Reproduction*, **21**, 2216–2222.

Royal College of Obstetricians and Gynaecologists (RCOG) (2011). The Investigation and Treatment of Couples with Recurrent Miscarriage. Green-Top Guideline 2011, No. 17, http://www.rcog.org.uk/ (accessed 21 June 2013)

NK Cells in Peripheral Blood and the Endometrium

Gavin Sacks[1,2,3]

[1] University of New South Wales, Sydney, NSW, Australia
[2] IVF Australia, Sydney, NSW, Australia
[3] St George Hospital, Sydney, NSW, Australia

Introduction

Investigations form the cornerstone of modern medicine. Without them, clinical practice based on anecdote and experience would be little different from services offered by many complementary practitioners. But, as all clinicians will know, investigations do not always identify a simple cause-and-effect relationship, and treatment based on them is not always certain to cure the problem. Indeed, such clinical interventions are relatively rare. Sometimes investigations provide insight to help patient understanding, or to guide clinical management. Sometimes the very act of doing them provides therapeutic benefit in terms of stress reduction or enhancing the doctor–patient relationship. In other words, while the ultimate purpose of an investigation must be to improve clinical outcome, and studies must strive to prove such a cause-and-effect relationship, clinical benefits may be more subtle.

Natural Killer (NK) cell testing for women with recurrent pregnancy loss is still an evolving science. Benefits are not yet proven, and some academics still argue strongly against it. They claim that there is no causal relationship yet demonstrated between NK test results and miscarriage, that peripheral blood testing can offer no insight into implantation immunology, that any benefit from intervention must be offset by the good prognosis many have without any intervention, and that there is a real danger that "desperate" women will be "taken advantage of" by the promise of illusionary diagnoses and treatments. It is important to understand these issues in order to counsel patients appropriately. And the relevance of NK cell testing must be understood in this context.

Recurrent Pregnancy Loss, First Edition. Edited by Ole B. Christiansen.
© 2014 John Wiley & Sons, Ltd. Published 2014 by John Wiley & Sons, Ltd.

PEARLS TO TAKE HOME

NK cell testing benefits:

1. May identify an immunological cause of recurrent miscarriage (15–25%)
2. May guide supportive therapy for next pregnancy (e.g., Progesterone or prednisolone)
3. Acknowledges patient concern with her immune system
4. Gives patient comfort that "everything" is being tested
5. Provides patient with confidence that her doctor is thinking broadly about her problem

---

NK cells and reproduction

There is no doubt that NK cells do have an important and perhaps critical role to play in the establishment of early pregnancy. Whilst NK cells are distributed widely in all tissues, they are especially concentrated in the uterus where they are the main immune cells present. Uterine (u)NK cell numbers increase enormously from 10% of stromal cells in the proliferative phase to 20% in the late secretory phase, and >30% in early pregnancy. In the absence of implantation, uNK cells undergo apoptosis that heralds menstruation.

NK cells are part of the innate and evolutionary older branch of the immune system and have a primary function of "immune surveillance." They do not require activation in order to kill cells that are missing "self" markers of major histocompatibility complex (MHC) class I, as in cells affected by intracellular infection or cancer. Since placental cells do not express classic MHC class I proteins except HLA-C (probably to avoid attack by maternal T cells), they are vulnerable to attack by NK cells instead. In theory, therefore, uNK cells may limit (or regulate) trophoblast (placental cell) invasion, by direct cytotoxicity or cytokine production. However, uNK cells have never been shown to be cytotoxic to trophoblast cells *in vivo*, and *in vitro* require coculture with interleukin (IL)-2 to induce cytotoxicity (not surprisingly, IL-2 is not usually present at the maternal–fetal interface).

It is likely that the majority of uNK cells are recruited directly from the peripheral blood pool of NK cells every month, and recent studies have suggested correlation between uNK and blood (b)NK cell numbers. However, the relationship between bNK cells and uNK cells is more complex. All NK cells are, by definition, lymphocytes, which are not T cells ($CD3^-$) and express the surface marker CD56. Two main subtypes exist. $CD56^{+Bright}$ express high-density CD56, are $CD16^-$, and produce cytokines (IFN-γ, TNF-β, IL-10, and GM-CSF). These represent 90% of uNK cells but only 10% of bNK cells. The other subtype, comprising 10% of uNK cells but 90% of bNK cells, are $CD56^{+Dim}$ NK cells, which express low-density CD56, are $CD16^+$, have limited cytokine output, and are primarily responsible for NK cell cytotoxicity. These two subtypes also express different activating receptors (CD69) and inhibiting receptors (killer immunoglobulin-like receptors (KIR) and CD94).

Methods of assessment

Much of the controversy surrounding NK cell analysis is largely the result of poor study design, overinterpretation of results, and little appreciation of the complexities of the laboratory methods used. In most published studies, the "patient" group is very heterogeneous; often including women with both recurrent miscarriage and repeated IVF failure (which themselves can have varied definitions). Controls are difficult to recruit (some studies have had no control group), and even more difficult to define. It is entirely plausible, for example, that a "fertile" woman may have future secondary reproductive failure.

The assessment of uNK cells can be done by flow cytometry but the isolation of the uNK cells for this procedure is technically extremely difficult. Therefore, assessment of uNK cells is normally done by immunohistochemistry, the subjectiveness and limitations of which are rarely appreciated. First of all, it is only possible to count CD56+ cells, without any measurement of subtype or level of activation. Thus, for example, high levels of CD56$^{+Bright}$ may reflect a very different immunological environment to high levels of CD56^{+Dim}. Second, the endometrium is a complex glandular histological structure, and counting cells in one area gives wildly different results to counting in another. It takes a considerable effort for a pathologist to develop a reliable and consistent method of counting. Most tests for uNK cells are performed at the time of the "implantation window." But uNK cell numbers vary enormously on a daily basis at that time, and interpretation of cell levels needs to be appropriate for that exact day of the cycle. Few laboratories will have sufficient data to be able to do that.

The main criticism for analysis of bNK cells is that they are mainly of different phenotype to the majority of uNK cells, and therefore cannot bear any useful relationship to uNK cell numbers, and in any case are far from the site of embryo implantation. But endometrial biopsy is an invasive and painful procedure, and the prospect of a blood test assessment of immunological dysfunction has significant appeal. Although the majority (90%) of uNK and bNK cells are of different phenotype, it is simply not known what changes in the ratio of subtypes may have on implantation. Thus, it is hypothesized that higher levels of activated CD56^{+Dim} bNK cells may lead to an altered phenotype ratio in the endometrium due to monthly recruitment. Alternatively, it is also possible that bNK cell activity represents a marker for some other (as yet undefined) immunological disorder. This marker may be nonspecific – in the same way as a raised white blood cell count or C-reactive protein level indicates the likelihood of infection somewhere in the body.

A number of assays have been used for the analysis of bNK cells, including the proportion of bNK cells out of all lymphocytes, concentration, surface markers of activation (flow cytometric analysis), and *in vitro* assays of biological activity. These methods are not necessarily correlated, and results may be potentially affected by venipuncture conditions and transport to the lab, protocols for preparation and labelling, and the gating of cell populations in flow cytometry analysis. Therefore considerable effort needs to be undertaken to standardise conditions before using an assay for research or clinical purposes, and comparisons with other studies need to take these factors into account. Although population studies demonstrate a wide reference range for bNK cells (3–31%), the corrected range for females is 5–20% (and this includes women with reproductive failure). There are also numerous other physiological variables that could affect bNK cell levels, including acute stress and exercise (increased), the menstrual cycle and IVF stimulation.

⚘ SCIENCE REVISITED

NK cell testing requires complex laboratory methodology that needs to be validated at a local level. Published studies must also be assessed against this background. Endometrial NK cell assessment is invasive and certainly requires a dedicated pathologist to provide reliable results. Blood NK cell assessment can potentially be performed by any hematology lab at a basic level. Our published studies (see Bibliography) indicate that 15–25% of women with RM have high NK cell levels.

NK cell analysis in recurrent miscarriage

Peripheral blood NK cell analysis in reproductive failure was first described in 1996 by Alan Beer's group in Chicago. In a poorly controlled study, it was famously claimed that high levels could be defined by bNK cell numbers >12%, and that no women with bNK levels over 18% had a successful pregnancy outcome, unless treated with immunoglobulin therapy. Other groups have since shown that in women with unexplained reproductive failure (including both those with RM and repeated IVF failure), bNK cells have higher preconceptual activity and cytotoxicity (^{51}Chromium-release assay), higher expression of the surface activation marker CD69, and lower expression of the inhibitory marker CD94. Women with raised NK cell activity have about a fourfold increase risk of miscarriage with karyotypically normal fetuses. In early pregnancy (including after IVF), lower levels of bNK cell cytotoxicity are significantly associated with live birth. One study showed that bNK cell cytotoxicity is higher in women with primary compared to those with secondary recurrent miscarriage.

In women with unexplained infertility, high bNK cell activity is associated with significantly lower conception rates over a 2-year follow-up. In the IVF setting, it has been claimed that lower bNK cell cytotoxicity on the day of embryo transfer is significantly associated with live birth. Another study used a receiver operating characteristic analysis to show that women undergoing IVF with raised CD69 expression on bNK cells had a significantly reduced implantation rate (13.1 vs. 28.2%), pregnancy rate (23.1 vs. 48.3%) and live birth rate (7.7 vs. 40.2%), and manifested a higher miscarriage rate (66.7 vs. 16.7%).

Given the invasive nature of uNK cell testing, there are fewer such studies in women with reproductive failure. However, numerous studies have similarly demonstrated that women with unexplained RM or repeated IVF failure have "high" uNK cell levels. Perhaps most significantly, it has been shown that preconceptual numbers are increased in women who subsequently have karyotypically normal miscarriages. Furthermore, a critical study using flow cytometry rather than immunohistochemistry showed that women with unexplained RM have increased uNK cells of the CD56^{+Dim} subtype. This supports the hypothesis that increased or activated bNK cells (primarily CD56^{+Dim} cells) alter the uNK cell subtype population, which may be in turn detrimental to successful implantation.

NK cell testing in practice

In one of the largest studies to date, work in Sydney has attempted to assess the reliability and establish reference levels for NK cell testing in women with RM. Endometrial biopsies were taken in the luteal phase (the time of implantation) and assessed by immunohistochemistry. It was immediately apparent that (i) the complexity of the tissue led to significant variability in cells counted (e.g., due to the presence of glands or cell clusters), and (ii) uNK cell numbers increased rapidly each day of the mid to late luteal phase. This new data challenges previous assumptions defining fixed reference ranges and illustrates two critical principals for uNK cell testing: (i) It requires a dedicated pathologist with an interest in this area in order to report reliable cell counts, and (ii) it requires a large database to provide daily reference ranges for a given population. It is clear that simply sending a sample to a general pathology laboratory is unlikely to produce any useful information on NK cell levels. Testing for uNK cells is still a highly specialized investigation that is only available in certain tertiary centers with a research interest in the topic.

Testing for bNK cells, on the other hand, has potential advantages and may be more widely available. In terms of a diagnostic test, a simple blood test is obviously far preferable to a uterine biopsy for the patient. The criticism that blood testing is irrelevant for assessment of events at implantation in the uterus ignores the facts that (i) in general medicine many blood tests gain information about distant organs, and (ii) numerous studies have shown high bNK cell levels in women with RM. Although our work in Sydney (and others elsewhere) has showed that high levels of bNK cells are strongly correlated with high levels of uNK cells, such a demonstration is more interesting from a research pathophysiological perspective than a clinical one. In reality, in comparison with uNK cell testing, bNK cell testing is an independent test, which uses different methodology (flow cytometry) on different cell types. In one of the largest and most detailed studies to date, we have shown that for bNK cells, the strongest discriminating factors (for nonpregnant women with RM vs. controls) are (i) the number of bNK cells expressed as a percentage of lymphocytes (normal <18%), and (ii) the concentration of activated CD56^{+Dim} bNK cells (determined with the CD69 marker; normal $<12 \times 10^6$/l). Flow cytometry is performed in all hospitals to varying degrees, and simple enumeration of bNK cell numbers (as a percentage of lymphocytes) should be possible in most large hematology labs. The CD69 marker test of bNK cell activation requires a dedicated flow cytometrist to perform labelling and gating. There are also important issues to take into account such as transport of specimens to the lab (time and shaking could affect bNK cell function), and protocols for fixation and labelling. In other words, just as is the case for uNK cell testing, bNK cell testing also requires the setting up of local systems and controls to obtain reliable results.

Using methods recently published, we have defined a population of 15–25% of women with unexplained RM as having "high" uNK cell levels, "high" bNK cell levels or activation, or both. It is not known why some women have higher levels than others, how or when their NK cell levels became raised. No longitudinal study has yet been done. Such a diagnosis is useful because of the association with RM, although it is certainly not proven that high NK cell levels are in themselves a cause of miscarriage. In normal pregnancy, it is well recognized that bNK cell levels and functional activity are suppressed, and this provides the rationale to attempt to suppress NK cell levels in women with known high levels and a clinical diagnosis of RM.

Targeted immune therapy

Immune therapy to try to reduce miscarriage rates has a long and chequered history. This is partly due to the legacy of Peter Medawar's classic 1950s paper in which pregnancy immunology was compared with a tissue transplant, and hence the need for maternal immune suppression. While more recent work has significantly refined that hypothesis, it is clear that NK cells are a critical part in the maternal recognition of a conceptus and establishment of the maternal–fetal interface. Animals with depleted NK cells do not have successful pregnancies. Implantation and pregnancy in general are inflammatory states, and it is hypothesized that the absence of inflammation can be just as detrimental as an excessive inflammatory state. So, can NK cell testing identify that subgroup of women with "excessive" immunological activity leading to a poor endometrial environment (e.g., abnormal local cytokine profile) and higher risk of miscarriage? Can such women be targeted for immune therapy?

A RCT to assess the effectiveness of immune therapy in women with high NK cell activity is urgently needed, and trials in the United Kingdom and Australia are currently being undertaken. At present, clinical guidance relies on less rigorous evidence. There have been a number of case reports, one of which described a woman with 19 successive miscarriages and high uNK cells who was successfully treated with prednisolone (at a dose that was shown to suppress uNK cell levels). A number of other observational studies have suggested benefit, although their interpretation is prone to possible bias. Options for immune therapy include prednisolone, dexamethasone, IVIG, intralipid, and anti-TNF-alpha. Heparin and even progesterone provide milder immune-suppressive effects and should be considered given their safety and cost. There is no NK specific drug and, given our current understanding of pregnancy immunology, no particular therapy is obviously preferable (immune therapies have never been compared in a single trial). Therapies should be regarded as experimental, with determining factors including cost, potential harm to mother and fetus, and availability.

In Sydney, having defined a population of women with RM who have high NK cell levels (by blood test or endometrial biopsy), empirical treatment is given in the form of prednisolone 20 mg daily. This is commenced as soon as the woman has a positive pregnancy test, and continued until 12 weeks gestation. In a population of women ($n = 87$) with a very poor prognosis (median age = 39, median number of miscarriages = 6 over 4 years of trying to conceive), in those treated with prednisolone for high NK cell levels, 52% had a live birth following treatment, 41% within a year, and the majority (66%) succeeded in their first pregnancy with immune therapy. Those who did not succeed were noted to have multiple miscarriage factors compared to the successful cases that were more likely to have "unexplained" RM (i.e., high NK cell levels only).

PATIENT ADVICE

On current evidence, it is reasonable to provide empirical therapy with progesterone and/or heparin first line. Both have mild NK-suppressive effects. A more powerful agent is prednisolone, which is commonly available and as effective at suppressing NK cells as other more expensive regimes (e.g., IVIG). Common side effects include insomnia and fluid retention. More severe potential maternal side effects such as diabetes, osteoporosis, and premature labor are extremely rare (never been reported) when given at moderate doses (20 mg daily) for the first trimester only. The only reported possible fetal side effect is cleft palate, although the incidence is also extremely rare.

Immune therapy caution

A key issue to take into account is the potential that immune therapy could do more harm than good. In the absence of randomized trials, it is of course impossible to be sure that immune therapy doesn't *reduce* overall success rates. That is a major reason to be particularly cautious in using immune therapy in women without a clinical diagnosis (e.g., in women who might have high NK cell levels but no history of miscarriage). Furthermore, therapy in early pregnancy has the potential to affect the fetus, and some effects may only be discovered some years later. The side effect profile and risks of immune therapy (for mother and fetus) need to be carefully weighed up and managed in any program offering NK cell testing. Ongoing studies and long-term follow-up are essential.

⚓ CAUTION

NK cell testing inevitably leads to the potential for immune therapy. Options in increasing order of strength are:

- progesterone
- heparin
- prednisolone/IVIG/intralipid/anti-TNF-alpha

Potential risks and side effects on both the fetus and mother need to be discussed with the patient. Therapy is unproven in this context, and no therapy is known to be superior. Therefore, use the safest, simplest, and cheapest first.

When to offer NK cell testing

As information has become so widely available, NK cell testing is almost impossible to ignore. Patients frequently discover the possibility of such testing on simple Internet searches or via patient forums. There is little point in doctors denying access to such testing on the basis that it is not yet proven to be effective. It may turn out to be impossible to actually prove that it is either effective or ineffective. Doctors would be best advised to understand the background (as discussed earlier), and take a progressive empirical approach with individualized care. What does this mean?

First of all, we must all be aware that many women are particularly concerned that their immune system is a problem. Women are prone to autoimmune conditions such as thyroid disease, and have an innate concern of their ability to carry a pregnancy. A survey in Sydney has found that nearly two-thirds of patients admitted using alternative therapies such as acupuncture and herbs. Such alternative practitioners have been successful as they acknowledge concern that a successful pregnancy requires complex whole body interactions, and this is barely assessed by conventional highly specific RM investigations such as karyotype and uterine morphology. For better or worse, NK cell testing is currently the most widely known and available test of the immune system, and as such offers a potential insight into the broader assessment of a woman's reproductive health. Some women request such testing at an early stage, and there is no reason to deny them if reliable NK testing is available. In Sydney, a blood test for NK cell analysis costs less than $100.

On current evidence, NK cell testing should not be offered as part of "routine" investigation for RM (defined as three or more miscarriages). However, if a reliable test is available, it should be done on request, or in more significant reproductive difficulty (e.g., five or more unexplained miscarriages, age over 36, IVF). Clearly, a blood test would be preferable, although on current evidence, optimal information is achieved with testing for both bNK and uNK cells. I do not believe that uNK cell testing by immunohistochemistry is a "better" test even though it samples the site of the problem (implantation). Flow cytometry offers significantly more detailed information on NK cell subtypes and activation status that may be more relevant. Also, flow cytometry for uNK cells is technically extremely difficult. Not many centers are able to offer both uterine and blood testing.

Interest in NK cell analysis has so far primarily been for patients with otherwise *unexplained* RM. It has been used as a means of exploring possibilities that are, by definition, at the frontiers of knowledge. We must be cautious in assuming that everyone with "unexplained RM" must have an "overactive" immune system. In Sydney, 15–25% of women with unexplained repeated reproductive failure have high NK cell levels (although a normal NK result does not exclude the possibility of an immune disorder). We must also remember that high NK cell levels may not be the cause of the problem – they may simply be associated with it. On the other hand, treatment with immune therapy (on an empirical basis) is not necessarily confined to women with high NK cells. So, what is the relevance of NK cell testing in women with RM?

NK cell testing offers the *potential* to target immune therapy to women who are more likely to benefit from it, and so may improve success rates. NK testing may be beneficial in other ways too. Many women appreciate the concept of looking for a cause of their infertility. It gives them confidence that their doctor is thinking and individualizing their problem. By acknowledging the importance of the immune system, it may reduce stress, and can give some patients the hope they need to keep trying.

Methodology is critical. Any test must be thoroughly validated and, in the absence of better-quality evidence, NK testing for targeted immune therapy should be done in the context of a trial. Patients should be advised of the experimental nature of the approach, and considerable caution should be undertaken to avoid the situation where marketing precedes the evidence. In that way, it is incumbent on us to push this frontier of reproductive medicine, rather than simply turn our back on it. Our patients expect nothing less.

★ **TIPS AND TRICKS**

In view of the lack of RCTs, an empirical, individualized approach to NK cell testing is recommended:

Offer testing (i) on request, (ii) after conventional miscarriage investigations have been found normal, (iii) after failure of conservative management or treatment of other miscarriage causes, (iv) after five or more unexplained miscarriages, (v) women over age 36, (vi) women with miscarriage after IVF.

Management of high NK cell levels must account for (i) strength of evidence for immune dysfunction (e.g., exact NK cell levels, whether information from just blood or uterine testing, reliability of labs, other autoimmune abnormalities), (ii) severity of clinical problem (e.g., number of miscarriages, requirement of IVF), (iii) immune therapy available, tolerable, and affordable.

The choice of immune therapy depends on how important the problem (high NK cells) is considered to be in relation to the risks, side effect, and cost of therapy

---

Bibliography

King, K., Smith, S., Chapman, M. and Sacks, G.P. (2010) Detailed analysis of peripheral blood natural killer (NK) cells in women with recurrent miscarriage. *Human Reproduction*, **25**, 52–58.

Rai, R., Sacks, G.P. and Trew, G. (2005) Natural killer cells in reproductive failure: theory, practice and prejudice. *Human Reproduction*, **20**, 1123–1126.

Russell, P., Anderson, L., Lieberman, D. *et al.* (2011) The distribution of immune cells and macrophages in the endometrium of women with recurrent reproductive failure I: Techniques. *Journal of Reproduction Immunology*, **91**, 90–102.

4

Cytokines and Cytokine Gene Polymorphisms in Recurrent Pregnancy Loss

Silvia Daher, Maria Regina Torloni and Rosiane Mattar

Department of Obstetrics, São Paulo Federal University (UNIFESP), São Paulo, SP, Brazil

Introduction – Cytokines and pregnancy: basic concepts

The immune paradox that enables the development of a successful pregnancy (SP) is still unsolved. A complex network of factors and mechanisms is involved in maternal–fetal interaction to ensure that the genetically incompatible fetus is protected from maternal immune response. Cytokines, nonantibody mediator proteins secreted by inflammatory leukocytes and some nonleucocytes cells, influence all steps of reproduction, playing a fundamental role in pregnancy outcome.

Different endometrial cells produce cytokines under the influence of hormones. Under normal circumstances, these mediators promote the growth and differentiation of trophoblasts; in certain cases they may also have an opposite effect, activating a maternal attack on trophoblasts. The pattern of local maternal response to trophoblast cells, that is, immune tolerance or immune stimulation, depends on the interaction between cytokines and cell surface receptors, but also on the specific type of mediator that is predominant and on its quantity.

The endometrial leukocyte population varies throughout the menstrual cycle; however, an impressive number of T-cells, uterine-NK (uNK) cells, and macrophages are always present. Human CD4 T-helper (Th) cells, a subpopulation of T cells, can be classified functionally into Th1, Th2, T regulatory (Tregs), and Th17 subsets (Figure 4.1). The Th1 subpopulation typically produces proinflammatory cytokines, including interleukin (IL)-2, tumor necrosis factor (TNF)-α, and interferon (IFN)-γ, and it is involved in cellular immunity and plays an important role against intracellular infections. In contrast, Th2 cells are anti-inflammatory, involved in humoral immunity, and produce IL-4, IL-5, IL-6, IL-9, IL-10, and IL-13. These two subsets, Th1 and Th2, are mutually inhibitory and modulated by Tregs. The Treg subpopulation secretes the transforming growth factor (TGF)-β and IL-10, as well as the forkhead box P3 (FoxP3) transcription factor.

More recent studies have demonstrated that under specific conditions, such as TGF-β stimulus in the presence of IL-6, CD4 T-helper cells may differentiate into

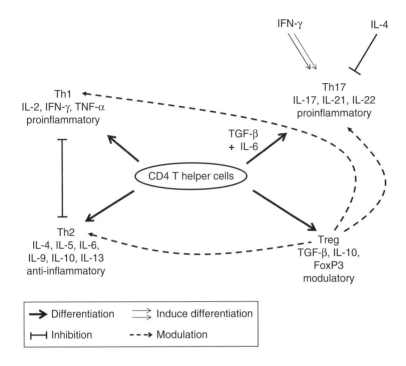

Figure 4.1 CD4 T cell subpopulations: cytokine profile and interactions.

another functional T-cell subset: Th17 cells. While IL-4 inhibits the development of Th17, IFN-γ and TGF-β induce the development of Th17 memory cells. These memory cells have the ability to respond to a re-encounter with a specific antigen more effectively than if at a first encounter. Evidence suggests that the Th17 subset is a potent inducer of inflammation, whereas Treg cells have a critical role for immunoregulation and in the induction of tolerance. The function of T cells (Th1, Th2, and Th17) is modulated by CD4+/CD25+ Treg cells.

By regulating the endometrial cytokine environment, T lymphocytes play a central role in preparing the implantation site, under the influence of gestational hormones.

An initial sterile inflammatory maternal immune response to the embryo is necessary for adequate implantation, angiogenesis, trophoblast invasion, and placental development. However, if it is not controlled, this immune response can be harmful for the embryo and/or the mother.

Several receptors of pro-inflammatory IL-1 mediators, such as IL-1β and IL-1, are expressed in endometrial and trophoblast cells. Evidence suggests that IL-1 is directly involved in implantation and that it is also a potent inducer of different mediators, including the leukemia inhibitory factor (LIF) and IL-6 in endometrial and trophoblast cells. Moreover, since IL-1 can stimulate Th2 cell generation, IL-1 may be involved in the regulation of Th1/Th2 cytokine production.

LIF and IL-11 have also been implicated in the implantation process. During pregnancy, LIF is expressed in villous and extravillous trophoblasts (EVTs) as well as in decidual leukocytes. Animal experiments and in vitro studies both using primary EVTs suggest that LIF mediates interaction between these two cell populations, exerting a central role in trophoblast invasion. Similarly, IL-11 and the IL-11 receptor (IL-11R) are intensely expressed in decidual cells during early pregnancy and seem to be involved in placentation according to animal and human *in vitro experiments*. Clinical data support this hypothesis since low levels of these cytokines have been detected in the endometrium of women with infertility and endometriosis. Similarly, low LIF and IL11 concentrations have been detected in uterine flushing of women with unexplained infertility or multiple implantation failures. Moreover, women with unexplained repeated pregnancy loss (RPL) have lower plasma IL11 than women with SPs.

Cytokine profile in healthy pregnancy and in RPL
One of the causes of RPL is thought to be impaired production of cytokines by maternal cells in response to fetal antigens. Transplant studies and experimental data suggest that SP depends on the development of a predominant Th2-type immunity profile, while an increase in Th1 cytokines has been associated with poor gestational outcomes.

The endometrial production of TNF-α varies throughout the menstrual cycle and also during gestation. Both IFN-γ and TNF-α seem to have a negative impact on pregnancy development. This abortive effect has been attributed to deficient tropho-blast invasion and placentation, and also to excessive activation of uNK cells and macrophages. In contrast, IL-4 and IL-10 favor pregnancy development by inhibiting Th1 cells and macrophage function. Accordingly, women with RPL have increased IFN-γ/IL-4, TNF-α/IL-4, and TNF-α/IL-10 ratios in their peripheral blood.

More recent studies contested the Th1/Th2 hypothesis and suggest that oversti-mulation of both profiles might be harmful to pregnancy development. A balance between Th1 and Th2 immunity mediators is determinant for adequate maternal and fetal interaction. It is important to emphasize that besides T lymphocytes, other cell types (such as NK cells, macrophages, dendritic cells, and trophoblast cells) also produce cyto-kines as well as other pro- and anti-inflammatory mediators at the maternal–fetal inter-face. Several factors, such as hormones, may favor the differentiation of Th cells into Th1 or Th2. Progesterone is a potent inducer of Th2 type subset, whereas relaxin and estradiol stimulate the development of IFN-γ and Th1 cells. Infection during pregnancy can also drive the immune response from an anti-inflammatory to an inflammatory profile.

The main challenge is to maintain an adequate level of inflammatory and anti-inflammatory mediators adjusted according to the different stages of reproduction. In an SP, trophoblast cells influence the cytokine profile, which can downregulate type 1 cytokine expressing NK and T cells. Moreover, trophoblast cells seem to be involved in the recruitment and activation of immune cells (Tregs and monocytes), in order to avoid an exacerbated inflammatory response at the local interface to avoid tissue damage and support embryo growth and survival.

Higher levels of Th2 cytokines (IL-6 and IL-10) have been detected in supernatants of peripheral blood mononuclear cultures (PBMC) from women with normal pregnan-cies in comparison with RPL patients. IL-10 seems to be the most potent immunosup-pressive and anti-inflammatory molecule. A key regulator of Th2 immune responses, IL-10, is an important antagonist for TNF-α and IFN-γ, and a major anti-inflammatory cytokine at the feto–placental interface. Pregnant women with a history of RPL who go on to have another miscarriage have more severe alterations than those with a similar history but who have a successful outcome.

The Th1 cytokine IFN-γ, especially in the presence of IL-2, IL-12, IL-15, and IL-18, is a potent inducer of NK cell proliferation, maturation, and activation. While these cells appear to be necessary for implantation, they can be harmful to the embryo when their number is excessive.

Despite having been considered harmful to gestation in the past, the development of a local and controlled Th1 response is essential for successful implantation as well as throughout the first trimester of pregnancy. According to several studies, women with repeated implantation failure have increased or suppressed Th1 endometrial immunity. In agreement with these findings, a pro-inflammatory immune response characterized by the expression of IL-1, TNF-α, IL-6, and IL-10, but reduced levels of IL-2 and IFN-γ has been detected immediately after implantation at the maternal–fetal interface in healthy pregnant women. Samples of endometrium obtained during the peri-implantation stage of the cycle and decidua fragments from both groups of women were analyzed using different technical approaches.

Interactions between Treg cells, Th17 cells, and cytokines and normal pregnancy and RPL

The current hypothesis, which replaces the Th1/Th2 paradigm, is that a balanced secretion of Th1/Th2/Th17 and T regulatory cytokines is essential for SP.

The Treg subset plays an important role in the control of maternal immune response to the fetus. During pregnancy, CD4+/CD25– Treg precursor cells differentiate into CD4+/CD25+ (functional?) Tregs in the presence of estradiol and TGF-β. The two types of Treg cells (i.e., natural and adaptive) have an anti-inflammatory action at the maternal–fetal interface. While natural Tregs exert their effects by secreting TGF-β and IL-10, the other Treg subset (adaptive) interacts with dendritic cells, inducing indoleamine 2,3-dioxygenase (IDO), and consequently reduces inflammation by interfering in tryptophan metabolism.

During the follicular phase of fertile women, the number of Tregs increases in parallel to estrogen serum levels. This subpopulation accumulates in the deciduas and represents 14% of decidual T cells. The number of these cells increases starting early in the first trimester, reaches a plateau in the second trimester, and declines in the postpartum period.

Patients with RPL have a different Treg profile, with lower levels of TGF-β and IL-2, together with an increased production of IL-6, leading to impaired number/function of the Treg subset. This is consistent with the finding that during the follicular and luteal phases, RPL patients usually have a smaller number of Tregs and also functionally deficient Tregs in comparison to women with SPs.

The number of Th17 cells apparently remains unchanged throughout pregnancy, although their numbers are usually higher in the decidua than in peripheral blood during the first trimester. Expansion of Th17 cells leading to increased secretion of inflammatory mediators has been associated with pregnancy loss. The relationship between the two cell subsets (Tregs and Th17) seems to affect pregnancy outcome, and an inverse profile has been reported both in peripheral blood and the deciduas of women with RPL. In this scenario, IL-6 is a central element since it blocks the development of Tregs, which could suppress an exaggerated Th1 immunity, but

Table 4.1 Cytokines Profile in Women with Successful Pregnancy (SP) versus Recurrent Pregnancy Loss (RPL)

	SP	RPL
Predominant Profile	Anti-inflammatory	Inflammatory
Local		
	↑ IL-10	↑ IL-6

	↓ TNF-α, IFN-γ
	  – Implantation
		↑ IL-2, TNF-α, TNF-β, IFN-γ
		  – Endometrium

	Treg/Th17 >1	Treg/Th17 <1
Peripheral blood		
	↑ IL-10	↓ IL-10
		↑ IL-2, TNF-α, TNF-β, IFN-γ, IL-6
		↑ IFN-γ/IL-4, TNF-α/IL-4, TNF-α/IL-10
		↑ TNF-α producing T CD3+/CD4+
		↑ IFN-γ/IL-4+ producing T CD3+/CD8+
		↓ TGF-β
	Treg/Th17 >1	Treg/Th17 <1
		↓ number and function Treg

induces the differentiation of Th17. Accordingly, a few studies have shown that patients with RPL usually have increased IL-6 and soluble IL-6 receptor serum levels.

Table 4.1 summarizes the most frequent between cytokines profile in successful versus RPL patients.

Cytokine gene polymorphisms and RPL – an overview

Certain cytokine gene polymorphisms might influence the level of cytokine production, and numerous studies have reported associations between cytokine gene polymorphisms, disease susceptibility, and/or different clinical features/outcomes of diseases. An example is the recognized association between variants in the IL-10 gene promoter and IL-10 serum levels in healthy Spanish population. In agreement with this finding, one of these IL-10 gene polymorphisms seems to be associated with susceptibility to gastric cancer.

Considering the potential role of cytokines in unexplained RPL, many investigators have performed studies to analyze the relationship between this condition and different cytokine polymorphisms.

Due to their recognized role in reproduction, polymorphisms in genes responsible for IL-6, IL-10, IFN-γ, and TNF-α production have been extensively investigated.

Different TNF-α gene functional polymorphisms (at position –238, –308, and –863 in the nucleotide sequence) have been investigated and, despite some conflicting results, most investigators did not find a significant association between any of these TNF-α gene polymorphisms and RPL or multiple implantation failures.

Genetic association studies are often limited by small sample sizes but meta-analyses can increase the precision of these estimates. However, several reviews and meta-analyses failed to identify any significant associations between RPL and polymorphisms in the IFN-γ (+874 T), IL-1β (–511 T), IL-6 (–174 G), or IL-10 (–1082 A, or –819 T, or –592 A) genes that are associated with altered cytokine production.

A few studies have found a possible association between some specific IL-1 and IL-1R gene polymorphisms and RPL. However, these results have not been confirmed by other investigators.

Similarly, there are no conclusive findings indicating a possible association between functional IL-6 gene polymorphisms and RPL. To further complicate these investigations, genetic polymorphisms in IL-6 gene are especially susceptible to ethnicity. Therefore, it is difficult to compare the results of different studies due to racial disparities in the included participants.

Despite a few initial positive results suggesting an association between IL-10 (–592C/A) gene polymorphisms and RPL, most of the studies that evaluated three different single nucleotide polymorphisms (SNPs) (1082G/A, 819C/T, 592C/A) could not confirm these findings. Similarly, several studies on TGF-β gene polymorphisms failed to find any association with RPL.

Only a few studies analyzed the relationship between genotype and phenotype in women with RPL. Most of the reports focused on genotype and alleles evaluation and did not assess gene expression. In addition, some investigators searched for a correlation between coding genes and biological expression but using a reduced number of samples and under specific conditions.

Up to the present, there is no evidence to support or recommend the evaluation of cytokine gene polymorphisms in the investigation of RPL or multiple implantation failure. Many of these polymorphisms have been evaluated only in isolated studies that enrolled a small number of patients. Furthermore, most of these studies were not confirmed by subsequent studies or were in fact refuted by other investigators. Other issues that may contribute to contradictory results in these studies include: (i) the possibility that other SNPs and also other factors may affect cytokine levels; (ii) differences in ethnic background, environmental factors, and participant selection criteria; and (iii) the possible effect of a combination of different cytokine gene polymorphisms on cytokine production and the occurrence of RPL.

Practical evaluation of cytokines for the diagnostic of RPL

A major problem in the study and evaluation of immune mediators in pregnancy relates to the inherent difficulty of assessing the maternal–fetal interface unit. While the implicated factors act locally, most of the studies have assessed these mediators systemically, on peripheral blood samples. Local abnormalities, both quantitative or functional, may go undetected in systemic evaluations. Additionally, there is no way to ensure that there is a correlation between local and systemic levels of cytokines. Therefore, the results of the available systemic (noninvasive laboratory) tests must be interpreted with caution, since they do not necessarily reflect the immunological events occurring at the maternal–fetal interface. Furthermore, it is important to differentiate between women with repeated implantation failure and those with RPL since the former are more severely immunologically compromised than the latter. The correlation between cytokine production in decidual lymphocytes and peripheral blood cells needs to be clarified before measurements of cytokine production can be introduced into clinical practice.

Some reproductive clinic includes in its RPL screening protocol a few tests to evaluate cytokines and the Treg subset. Most of these centers assess the profile of cytokines produced in vitro, using stimulated T cells. Despite some variations, most of these centers analyze intracellular cytokine production. One of the most frequently used tests is the *Th1 and Th2 Intracellular Cytokine Assay, which assesses IL-6, TNF-α, and IFN-γ levels.* As previously reported, patients with RPL usually tend to have a Th1 profile. Outside of pregnancy, women with RPL and multiple implantation failures have significantly higher absolute cell counts of TNF-α expressing CD3+/CD4+ cells, and IFN-γ/IL-4 producing CD3+/CD8+ T-helper cell ratios than those of nonpregnant fertile women.

Another test sometimes used in RPL patients is the evaluation of Treg cells in endometrial biopsy tissues and in peripheral blood. Women with failed implantation or with early miscarriage seem to have a significant reduction of Foxp3 expressing Treg cells.

According to the most recent American College of Obstetricians and Gynecologists, Royal College of Obstetricians and Gynecologists, American Society for Reproductive Medicine, and Dutch Society of Obstetrics and Gynecology guidelines for the evaluation and management of RPL, up to the present there is insufficient evidence to support the inclusion of the evaluation of cytokines and cytokine gene polymorphisms in routine workups of all RPL patients.

Conclusion

Based on the best available current evidence, the evaluation of cytokines and cytokine gene polymorphisms should not be part of routine RPL workups and are not recommended by any of the major international obstetric guidelines. Up to the present, there is no evidence indicating that these tests will add any consistent information to the diagnostic and therapeutic strategies of patients with unexplained RPL.

⚛ SCIENCE REVISITED

The initial hypothesis that Th type 1 cytokines with proinflammatory effects such as IFN-γ, IL-2, and TNF-α are harmful and anti-inflammatory Th type 2 cytokines such as IL-4 and IL-10 are beneficial for pregnancy has recently been modified.

It is now believed that an adequate level of inflammatory and anti-inflammatory mediators adjusted according to the different stages of reproduction is important for successful implantation and placentation.

✋ CAUTION

The production of cytokines from decidual lymphocytes is strongly affected by female sex hormones such as progesterone and estradiol, and results of measurement of cytokines in the uterus or blood are therefore expected to be dependent on time in a menstrual cycle or stage of pregnancy.

PEARLS TO TAKE HOME

Certain cytokine gene polymorphisms might influence cytokine production.

The relationship between cytokine gene polymorphisms and recurrent pregnancy loss has only been evaluated in small studies.

Combination of such studies in meta-analyses is complicated by the fact that the levels of cytokines may be determined by combinations of several genes and that the prevalence of the genetic polymorphisms varies between different ethnic groups.

Bibliography

Bansal, A.S. (2010) Joining the immunological dots in recurrent miscarriage. *American Journal of Reproductive Immunology*, **64**, 307–315.

Choi, Y.K. and Kwak-Kim, J. (2008) Cytokine gene polymorphisms in recurrent spontaneous abortions: a comprehensive review. *American Journal Reproductive Immunology*, **60**, 91–110.

Pan, F., Tian, J., Pan, Y.Y. and Zhang, Y. (2012) Association of IL-10-1082 promoter polymorphism with susceptibility to gastric cancer: evidence from 22 case-control studies. *Molecular Biology Reports.*, **39**, 7143–7154.

Saini, V., Arora, S., Yadv, A. and Bhattacharjee, J. (2011) Cytokines in recurrent pregnancy loss. *Clinica Chimica Acta*, **412**, 702–708.

Suárez, A., Castro, P., Alonso, R. *et al.* (2003) Interindividual variations in constitutive interleukin-10 messenger RNA and protein levels and their association with genetic polymorphisms. *Transplantation*, **75**, 711–717.

5

How to Assess the Prognosis after Recurrent Miscarriage

Howard J.A. Carp

Department of Obstetrics and Gynecology, Sheba Medical Center, Tel Hashomer & Tel Aviv University, Tel Hashomer, Israel

Introduction

A patient with recurrent pregnancy loss (RPL) usually requires four answers, the cause of her miscarriages, the prognosis both for the next pregnancy and whether she will ever have a live child, and what treatment can be offered to prevent a recurrence. The prognosis is a difficult question to answer. The classical approach has been to treat all patients with three or more miscarriages as one homogeneous group. Using this approach the prognosis for a subsequent live birth has been quoted to be approximately 60% after three miscarriages or 80% after two miscarriages. This relatively good prognosis in nontreated patients has made it almost impossible to show efficacy for any regimen of treatment, and has produced an approach that the relatively good prognosis indicates that treatment is not required unless demonstrated in randomized trials. The relatively good prognosis has been quoted in guidelines by the Royal College of Obstetricians and Gynaecologists, the American College of Obstetrics and Gynecology, and the European Society for Human Reproduction and Embryology. However, the converse is also true. Forty per cent of patients with three miscarriages will suffer a fourth miscarriage. After four miscarriages, the prognosis for a live birth is 46%, and 54% will miscarry again. Therefore, 22% (40% × 54%) of patients with three miscarriages will have two further miscarriages. In the author's series, after five pregnancy losses, the chance of a live birth is only 29%. Therefore accurate determination of prognosis is required.

PATIENT ADVICE

Patients with RPL are not a homogeneous group. The prognosis varies in various patients.

Patients want to know the chance of a live birth in the next pregnancy and if they will ever have a live child.

> **⚙ SCIENCE REVISITED**
>
> Overall prognosis for a live birth is 60% in patients with three miscarriages.
>   The only proven cause of miscarriage is embryonic chromosomal aberrations.
> All other "causes" are only associations.

Although the overall prognosis for a live birth has been quoted to be 60%, the prognosis is unknown in recurrent biochemical pregnancies, after in vitro fertilization, antiphospholipid syndrome (APS), or in the older woman. Various predictive factors have been reported to affect the prognosis, viz.: (i) The number of previous pregnancy losses. As the number of previous losses increases, the chance of a live birth decreases. Each subsequent miscarriage has been reported to lower the live birth rate by 24%. (ii) Maternal age. An older woman has a worse prognosis for a live birth. (iii) The karyotype of previous miscarriage. The patient with an aneuploid abortion has a better chance of a live birth (see Figure 5.1). (iv) Concurrent infertility. This has often been quoted as the time taken to conceive, or the need for infertility treatment. The patient with concurrent infertility has a poorer prognosis than the patient who conceives easily. (v) Early or late pregnancy losses, as the patient with late losses tends to have a worse prognosis. (vi) Primary, secondary, or tertiary aborter status has been reported to affect the prognosis, with the secondary aborter having a better prognosis than the primary or tertiary aborter. Primary aborters are defined as those who miscarry all their pregnancies, whereas secondary aborters may have had one or more pregnancies develop past 20 weeks. We define a third group known as tertiary aborters. These women have miscarriages, a live birth, and a further series of miscarriages.

> **⚙ SCIENCE REVISITED**
>
> Predictive factors for a live birth include:
>   The number of previous pregnancy losses, maternal age, karyotype of previous miscarriage, concurrent infertility, early or late pregnancy losses, primary, secondary, or tertiary aborter status, parental chromosomal rearrangements, antiphospholipid antibodies (aPL), hereditary thrombophilias, inappropriate immune responses, thyroid dysfunction, uterine anomalies, sperm defects, and psychological stress.

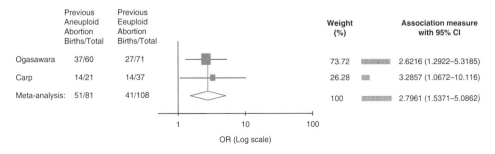

Figure 5.1 Effect of embryonic karyotype on live birth chance in subsequent pregnancy.

Additionally, there are a number of risk factors which may be related to cause. These include: (i) parental chromosomal rearrangements, (ii) aPL, (iii) hereditary thrombophilias, (iv) inappropriate immune responses, as shown by antipaternal complement dependent antibodies (APCA), and numbers and killing activity of natural killer (NK) cells, (v) thyroid dysfunction, (vi) uterine anomalies, (vii) sperm defects, (viii) psychological stress, etc. All of these may affect the subsequent prognosis for a live birth.

Many years ago, our team analyzed the clinical presentation of the first 489 patients with three or more miscarriages presenting to our service. Of these patients, 58% were primary aborters with no previous live births, 32% were secondary aborters, and 10% were tertiary aborters (miscarriages followed by a live birth and a further string of miscarriages). Moreover, 89% of losses were in the first trimester, 78% of abortuses were blighted ova, and 31% of patients had five or more abortions. We followed this population prospectively. There was a 45% subsequent live birth rate in the subsequent pregnancy without treatment. We reported that increasing the proportion of secondary aborters, the proportion of APCA positive patients, or the proportion of patients with only three miscarriages would have raised the live birth rate, making it reach 60% or even higher. If a patient has a mixed pattern of pregnancy losses with each loss having a different presentation, for example, blighted ovum followed by a second trimester loss of a live fetus, then a missed abortion, the cause is more likely to be due to chance than a recurrent cause, and her prognosis for a live birth will be good.

In a recent landmark publication Li *et al.* demonstrated some of the problems of interpreting the reports on prognosis of RPL, viz: RPL is most often defined as three or more consecutive losses. However, the American definition of two or more losses has led some investigators to include patients with two miscarriages in their series. Other series include nonconsecutive losses. Some investigators only include patients with first trimester miscarriages. Again the American definition of a miscarriage as a pregnancy lost prior to 20 weeks has led to the inclusion of the mid-trimester losses in some series.

SCIENCE REVISITED

Different series use different definitions of RPL, have different patient criteria, and quote the prognosis in different ways.

Furthermore, the prognosis varies in pregnancy as the pregnancy advances. The prognosis improves after fetal cardiac activity is detected in patients with multiple miscarriages of blighted ova. The prognosis similarly improves after the second trimester is reached. However, these criteria are not relevant for the relatively small number of patients who repeatedly lose pregnancies in the mid-trimester.

After the pregnancy succeeds, and the pregnancy reaches the third trimester, the pregnancy is at a higher risk of various obstetric complications. These are discussed in Chapter 11. They have previously been summarized by the author.

Method of study

Various methods have been used to assess the prognosis. Alberman in a landmark article asked female doctors to report on the outcome of previous pregnancies.

Pregnancies were classified according to gravidity. Seven hundred and forty-two women had had three previous pregnancies, 355 women had four previous pregnancies. Fourteen women had had three or more pregnancy losses. Of the 14 women with three losses, 10 became pregnant a fourth time, and six (60%) had a live birth. This study gave a good estimate of the prognosis. As the study consisted of physicians, delayed menstruation, induced abortions, ectopic pregnancies, and miscarriages were unlikely to be misclassified. However, there were no patients of gravidity five or higher. Therefore, there was no information on higher numbers of miscarriages.

Brigham *et al.* (1999) used a different approach. Seven hundred and sixteen women with a history of two or more consecutive miscarriages attending a dedicated miscarriage clinic were entered into a constantly updated database over a 10 year period. The prognosis was assessed for patients with idiopathic recurrent miscarriage (RM). Known associations of RPL such as aPL, oligomenorrhea, cervical incompetence, parental chromosomal rearrangements, second trimester loss, and patients treated for an abnormal finding were excluded from the study. A successful outcome was regarded as survival beyond 24 weeks. Ectopic pregnancies and termination of pregnancy in the subsequent pregnancy were excluded from the study sample. Of the 716 patients in the database, 222 had "idiopathic RM," conceived intrauterine pregnancies and were followed up. Also, 167 of the 222 patients (75%) had a successful outcome with survival beyond 24 weeks. This paper indicates a relatively good prognosis, but suffers from serious drawbacks. Twenty-four per cent of patients had only two miscarriages; there was no assessment of fetal chromosomal rearrangements. Twenty-three patients were lost to follow up. A live birth rate of 75% is quoted. However, 76 patients had no further pregnancies, two ectopic pregnancies, two terminations of pregnancies, and the live birth rate should be 167/302, that is, 55%.

Lund *et al.* (2012) used a cohort study with register-based follow-up at a tertiary center for investigation and treatment of RM in Denmark. Between 1986 and 2008, 1312 patients were enrolled. Patients with two miscarriages, non-Danish citizens, patients with insufficient information to confirm their previous pregnancy history, or patients with nonconsecutive miscarriages were excluded. The final study group consisted of 987 patients. Details of live birth, migration, death, or end of follow-up (June 30, 2010) were obtained from National Health Registers. The 987 women in the study group gave birth to 665 children (67%). This means that a full one-third of women did not achieve a live birth. When the figures were analyzed for maternal age, only 41.7% in women aged 40 years or older achieved a live birth within 5 years after the first consultation, compared to 81.3% of women aged 20–24 years at the time of first consultation. There was also a significant overall difference in the chance of a live birth according to the number of previous miscarriages. Compared to 50.2% of women with six or more previous miscarriages, 71.9% of women with three miscarriages achieved a live birth within 5 years of the first consultation. Note that 45% of women with six or more miscarriages never achieved a live birth. However, a major weakness of Lund *et al.*'s (2012) study is that the results were not corrected for treatment of specific causative factors.

Specific causes of RPL and prognosis

Number of Miscarriages

The number of previous miscarriages is probably the most important prognostic variable for a subsequent live birth. The prognosis for a subsequent live birth decreases with increasing numbers of miscarriages. Each subsequent miscarriage has been reported to lower the live birth rate by 24%. In multivariate analyses of clinical and paraclinical parameters of prognostic significance, the number of previous miscarriages has been reported as the strongest prognostic parameter even after adjustment for other risk factors. In Li et al.'s series, the live birth rate gradually dropped from 64% among women with two previous miscarriages to 43.2% among women with six or more miscarriages. In Lund et al.'s (2012) series 35% of patients with five miscarriages and, as stated earlier, 45% of patients with six or more miscarriages never achieved a live birth.

> ✋ **CAUTION**
>
> The number of previous miscarriages is the most important prognostic factor. Thirty-five per cent of patients with five miscarriages and, as stated earlier, 45% of patients with six or more miscarriages never achieved a live birth.

The incidence of chromosomal aberrations also decreases with increasing numbers of pregnancy losses. Thus, the patient with a larger number of pregnancy losses has a lower chance of an abnormal fetus and, hence, will benefit more from treatment for maternal causes of RPL. However, there are relatively few patients with a large number of miscarriages available for analysis. At the Sheba Medical Centre RPL clinic, approximately 30% of new referrals have five or more miscarriages compared to 19% of the patients in the international registry of the RM immunotherapy trialists group. However, there are only isolated reports of patients with five or more RPLs. Kwak et al. described the prevalence of aPL and antinuclear antibody according to gravidity. The prevalence of both antibodies increased from 34% in women with three pregnancy losses to 50% in gravidity five women. Kilpatrick and Liston have described 26 patients with five or more miscarriages, and calculated that the chance of five miscarriages occurring by chance is only 5% as opposed to 48% in women with three or more RPLs.

Maternal Age

Maternal age has been shown repeatedly to impact on pregnancy outcome. In the older age groups, fertility also falls with the approach of the menopause. Therefore, many women in the over 40s will never achieve a live birth. In Lund et al.'s (2012) series, 45% of women over the age of 40 with RM never achieved a live birth. The higher incidence of miscarriage could be the result of an age related increase in aneuploid conceptions, decreasing hormonal function, or cumulative exposure to unknown factors. In the author's series in which the abortus was karyotyped after three or more miscarriages, there was a 29% prevalence of embryonic chromosomal aberrations. This figure was 63% in women above the age of 40. In Sullivan *et al.*'s (2004) series, there was a 50% prevalence of aneuploid embryos in recurrently miscarrying women, compared to only 24% in the 20s and early 30s.

Karyotype of Previous Miscarriage

> **PATIENT ADVICE**
>
> Previous embryonic aneuploidy improves the prognosis for the subsequent pregnancy.
>   Fetal karyotyping should be performed for an accurate diagnosis and to determine the prognosis.

Embryonic chromosomal aberrations are the only definitive cause of miscarriage. All other so-called "causes" of miscarriage are in fact risk factors which are associated with a poorer prognosis. Fetal karyotyping has been recommended in a guideline for the Management of RPL by the Royal College of Obstetricians in the United Kingdom. However, the embryo is not karyotyped in most centers. Indeed, the value of fetal karyotyping has been hotly debated. Karyotyping the abortus allows the patient to be given prognostic information regarding subsequent pregnancy outcomes. Warburton and coworkers summarized 273 women who had had abortuses karyotyped. They concluded that after a previous trisomic miscarriage, the prognosis is favorable. Two subsequent studies have assessed the prognosis of the subsequent pregnancy according to the karyotype of the miscarriage. Patients with an aneuploid abortion have a better prognosis (see Figure 5.1). In women with three miscarriages and an aneuploidic miscarriage, reassurance of a good prognosis may be sufficient and may save the patient more extensive investigations and treatment of dubious value. This may not be the case in euploidic abortions. However, repeat aneuploidy has been estimated to occur in approximately 15% of patients after one aneuploid miscarriage. Consequently, 85% of patients with an aneuploid abortion can be assured that the prognosis is good and that the aneuploid abortion may be a chance occurrence. However, the other 15% may have a recurring cause of fetal aneuploidy, and can be offered pregestational screening diagnosis (PGS).

Concurrent Infertility

Concurrent infertility has been reported to occur between pregnancies in 32% of RPL. A history of infertility has been reported to result in a fourfold increase in risk of miscarriage. Logistic regression analysis of predictive factors in RM, showed that an increase of the subfertility index by 10 points decreased the odds for a successful pregnancy by 40%. In the author's series, 74 RPL patients (of 2316) were referred for assisted reproductive technology (ART) for subsequent infertility. Additionally, we have seen 182 ART patients who were referred due to RPL after ART (out of 2316). As stated earlier, the patient would want to know the prognosis in the subsequent pregnancy and whether she will ever have a live child. If she fails to conceive, the prognosis is obviously poor. Most studies on prognosis have not taken infertility into account.

The appearance of infertility after RPL with previously normal fertility is multifactorial. We need to ask whether the causes of infertility cause RPL, or whether the causes of RPL cause infertility (see Chapter 12). Both RPL and infertility may be due to chromosomal aberrations in the embryo. The abnormally thin endometrium causes infertility, but its effect on RPL has hardly been investigated. Additionally, many women with RPL undergo repeat curettage, a procedure which in itself may denude the endometrium, leading to adhesions, and loss of receptivity, subsequent infertility, and a poor prognosis both for conception and a live birth.

> **PATIENT ADVICE**
>
> Concurrent infertility worsens the prognosis.
> Repeated late pregnancy losses are associated with a worse prognosis.

Late Pregnancy Losses

Most studies on RPL have grouped both early and late losses together as a homogeneous group. However, the mechanism may be quite different. Early losses may be due to chromosomal aberrations in a large proportion of cases. The prevalence of chromosomal aberrations in late pregnancy losses is significantly less. Mid-trimester losses affect less patients than first trimester losses. The prevalence of late pregnancy losses has been reported to vary between 11% and 25% in different series. The patient with late losses tends to have a worse prognosis for later obstetric complications. Additionally, there is less likelihood of embryonic sporadic chromosomal aberrations.

Primary, Secondary, or Tertiary Aborter Status

In the author's series, the secondary aborter has a better prognosis than the primary or tertiary aborter. However, this finding has not been universal. Others have reported that the presence of a live birth does not alter the prognosis. The discrepancy between the interpretation of a previous live birth as a prognostic factor may be due to some studies combining secondary abortions and tertiary abortion into a single group. Additionally, some studies define secondary RPL as RPL after a live birth, others use gestational week 28 or 20 as the cutoff point.

Parental Chromosomal Rearrangements

Although the abortus is not often karyotyped, it is common practice to karyotype the parents. Indeed parental karyotyping is recommended in all guidelines on the management of RPL. However, parental karyotyping seeks balanced translocations and inversions rather than the more common numerical aberrations such as trisomy. Parental karyotypic aberrations have been found in 3–10% of couples with RM.

> **SCIENCE REVISITED**
>
> Parental karyotyping does not make a diagnosis or determine prognosis.
> In parental chromosomal aberrations, the embryo should be karyotyped to reach an accurate diagnosis.

Table 5.1 Subsequent Live Births in the Presence of Parental Chromosomal Aberrations

	Carp *et al.*	Goddijn *et al.*	Stephenson and Sierra	Ogasawara *et al.*	Total
Pregnancies	75	42	58	47	222
Live births	33	30	41	15	119
Proportion live births	44%	70%	71%	32%	53.6%
Mean no. of miscarriages	4.23	3.9	5.4	2.9	4.19

The problem is that parental karyotyping does not seem to be prognostic for subsequent pregnancies. Four studies have looked at the subsequent live birth rate in patients with RM and parental chromosomal rearrangements. These are summarized in Table 5.1. When the figures were combined, the live birth rate was 53.6% for patients with a mean of 4.19 previous miscarriages. This live birth rate of 53.6% is the expected rate for patients with four miscarriages, according to numerous series in the literature.

Patients are often advised that the presence of a parental karyotypic aberration diagnoses the cause of the miscarriage, as the aberration may be transmitted to the embryo in an unbalanced form. However, the author's team has examined the karyotype of abortuses from parents with karyotypic aberrations. Thirty-nine abortuses from recurrently miscarrying couples with parental karyotypic aberrations were karyotyped. Of the 39 embryos, 17 (44%) were euploid. Another 10 (26%) had the same balanced translocation as the parent. Hence, 70% were chromosomally normal. Only five (13%) abortuses had unbalanced translocations, whereas seven (18%) of the abortuses had subsequent abortuses with numerical aberrations unrelated to the parental chromosomal disorder (five trisomies and two embryos with monosomy X). Hence, in parental chromosomal aberrations, the embryo should be karyotyped to reach accurate diagnosis.

Antiphospholipid Antibodies

As parental karyotyping, testing for aPL is recommended in all guidelines on the management of RPL. However, there is no good cohort study on the natural history of RPL in the presence of aPL. The subsequent probability of a live birth can best be estimated from the placebo arm of studies on the effect of aspirin in the presence of RPL. In placebo-controlled trials the ascertainment of pregnancies is generally better than in nonrandomized studies since the patients are included according to a strict protocol and are more closely monitored in early pregnancy. There are three papers which have compared the use of aspirin to placebo, all three have been combined in a meta-analysis. Of 61 of pregnancies, 52 (85.2%) developed normally in the placebo group. However, it must be borne in mind that the four trials may have used different criteria for the laboratory diagnosis of aPl. Hence, there may be a subgroup of women with aPL who may not need anticoagulant or antiplatelet therapy.

> ⬡ **SCIENCE REVISITED**
>
> APS should be distinguished from aPL.
>   In RPL with aPL 85.2% of pregnancies developed normally in the placebo group with no treatment.

It may therefore be necessary to separate the mere occurrence of aPL from APS according to clinical criteria. aPL associated pregnancy loss seems to be associated with missed abortions in which a fetal heart was previously detected and losses at later stages of pregnancy than women with unexplained RPLs. In first trimester pregnancy losses, particularly those which present as blighted ova, the role of aPL is less clear, particularly as 30% of first trimester miscarriages are due to major chromosomal rearrangements in the presence of aPL. Moreover, APS is an autoimmune disease; in women with the full blown syndrome with previous thromboses, and autoimmune phenomena, the incidence of pregnancy loss is high. The serum from women with APS is highly teratogenic to rat embryos in culture, affects embryonic growth, and the purified IgG fraction of APS sera directly affect the embryo and yolk sac, reducing their growth.

Hereditary Thrombophilias

Genetic tendencies to thrombosis (hereditary thrombophilias) have been reported to predispose to thrombosis in decidual vessels, leading to fetal anoxia and possibly pregnancy loss. The hereditary thrombophilias include: antithrombin deficiency, protein C deficiency, protein S deficiency, activated protein C resistance, and factor V Leiden (FVL), homozygosity for the methylenetetrahydrofolate reductase mutation (MTHFR), C677T, and the prothrombin gene (FII) mutation G20210. In the presence of antithrombin, protein C, protein S, or FVL, the odds ratios for fetal loss after 28 weeks of gestation have been reported to be 5.2, 2.3, 3.3, and 2.0, respectively; the odds ratio was 14.3 for women with more than one type of inherited thrombophilia. Hereditary thrombophilias have also been reported to be associated with an increased risk of early fetal loss (less than 25 weeks) in women with protein C, protein S, or antithrombin deficiencies, and in FVL. The question then arises as to whether thrombophilias are more prevalent in women with RPL. The author has not found an increased prevalence of FVL, G20210A, or MTHFR in women with RMs. However, a recent meta-analysis of 31 case control studies has shown a significant association between hereditary thrombophilias and pregnancy loss.

> ⬡ **SCIENCE REVISITED**
>
> Hereditary thrombophilias are genetic tendencies to thrombosis, they do not necessarily cause thrombosis.

There are five studies examining the true incidence of pregnancy complications in the presence of thrombophilias and RPL. Two papers reported no increased subsequent miscarriage rate for patients with decreased protein C or S activity, or antithrombin.

FVL, G20210A or MTHFR. However, two papers have reported a lower live birth rate in women with the FVL mutation, and Lund *et al.* (2012) found a lower odds ratio for live birth in FVL and the prothrombin gene (G20210A) mutation. Salomon *et al.* (2004) have followed up 191 thrombophilic patients who attended an ultrasound clinic to prospectively assess obstetric complications. The blood flow to the fetus was not found to be compromised. Therefore, it seems that hereditary thrombophilias do impact on the prognosis of RPL but there is an urgent need for large prospective studies on the association of thrombophilia and miscarriage. However, the trial will need to control for number of previous miscarriages, maternal age, early or late miscarriages, and the confounding effects of embryonic chromosomal aberrations.

Immunological Factors

There is much evidence that aberrant maternal immune responses may lead to pregnancy loss. In the case of autoimmunity, the action of aPL is known and discussed earlier. During the years, numerous attempts have been made to find markers of an aberrant immune response. Sharing of human leukocyte antigens (HLAs) between both parents was thought to be a marker, as was decreased recognition in the missed lymphocyte reaction. The production of maternal alloantibodies directed against paternal/fetal HLAs was also thought to be a marker for an improved prognosis, and still carries some prognostic significance for patients with large numbers of miscarriages. These antibodies are not pathological, and seem to be produced with increased gestation.

> **PATIENT ADVICE**
>
> The markers of immunological mediated miscarriage remain to be accurately determined.

More recently, the presence of increased numbers and killing activity of large granular lymphocytes (LGL) bearing the CD56 antigen (also known as natural killer or NK cells) has been reported to be predictive of a poor prognosis in RPL. However, there has been doubt whether the number or killing activity reflects killing activity in the endometrium. The alterations in cellular immunology have also been examined in the endometrium and decidua. Around the time of implantation, approximately 20% of endometrial stroma cells are leukocytes, of which the majority are LGL. However, the endometrial LGL express a different set of surface markers to peripheral blood LGL. It is therefore uncertain whether measurement of peripheral blood LGL reflects the local situation in the endometrium. At present, peripheral blood NK cells are often taken as markers of a poor prognosis or an immunologically mediated miscarriage. However, there is no standardization of NK testing. NK numbers and activity are dependent on the method of assay, whether whole blood or fractionated mononuclear cells are used in the assay, the time of day, physical exercise, parity, and whether the samples have been previously frozen. There is also no agreed cutoff for determining immunologically mediated miscarriages.

Thyroid Dysfunction

Although hyperthyroidism has been associated with poor pregnancy outcomes, including preterm delivery, abruptio placentae, maternal heart failure, fetal growth restriction, and stillbirth, hyperthyroidism has not been reported commonly as an independent cause of RPL. Hypothyroidism is associated with infertility, both by impacting on oocytes at the level of the granulosa and luteal cells and inhibiting ovulation. Severe hypothyroidism rarely complicates pregnancy because of associated anovulation and infertility. However, in mild hypothyroidism, pregnancies can occur and are associated with higher rates of pregnancy loss and maternal complications. However, there is little evidence for a causal role.

Several studies have found an association between spontaneous abortions and autoantibodies to the thyroid gland, such as antithyroid peroxidase (TPO) or antithyroglobulin (Tg) antibodies. As thyroid dysfunction is not always detected in the presence of thyroid autoantibodies, the higher miscarriage rate in women with autoimmune thyroiditis could be due to the autoantibodies rather than an impaired hormonal state, or inability to meet the increased demand for thyroid hormones in early pregnancy. Other studies have not demonstrated an association between the presence of thyroid antibodies and pregnancy loss, and therefore the direct role of thyroid autoantibodies in fetal loss is debatable. The author has carried out a multicenter study of autoantibodies in reproductive failure. There was no higher prevalence of antithyroid antibodies (ATA) in RPL. Additionally, the author has followed up 298 women with a mean of 3.96 previous miscarriages. Sixty-nine were positive for TPO and/or Tg antibodies, compared to 229 who were negative for these ATA. Forty-six per cent of ATA positive women had a subsequent live birth (13/28) compared to 32% (25/78) of ATA negative women (RR = 1.55, CI 0.83–2.91). Therefore, the prognostic value of thyroid autoantibodies remains uncertain (see Chapter 2).

Uterine Anomalies

Anatomic uterine defects including diethylstilbestrol (DES) exposure, bicornuate and septate uterus, etc. have long been associated with RM. Using newer imaging modalities, it is currently estimated that the incidence of uterine anomalies in the general population is approximately 1%, and about threefold higher in women with RPL and poor reproductive outcomes. In a recent case controlled study of 1570 patients with two or more miscarriages there were only 25 live births in 42 patients (59.5%) in the women with uterine anomalies compared to 1096 births in 1528 (71.7%) in the control group with no uterine anomalies (p = 0.084).

> **⚖ SCIENCE REVISITED**
>
> Uterine anomalies impact on the progression of normal pregnancies, and must be considered to be a prognostic sign.

Additionally, the patients with uterine anomalies tended to lose euploid embryos, 15.4% of the miscarriages were aneuploid compared to 57.5% of the control patients (p = 0.006). Hence, uterine anomalies seem to impact on the progression of normal pregnancies, and must be considered a prognostic sign. In addition to pregnancy loss, uterine malformations predispose women to other reproductive difficulties including infertility, preterm labor, and abnormal fetal presentation.

Sperm Defects

Studies using conventional semen analysis showed that the male partners of women with RPL were not significantly different from control subjects. Hence, there is little value in performing a routine semen analysis. A study comparing 15 male partners of patients with RM with 10 controls and found no significant differences in their rate of sperm chromosomal hypohaploidy and hyperhaploidy. However, they reported a high incidence of chromosomal breaks and acentric fragments in the RM group. A significant increase in sex disomy in the spermatozoa of male partners of women with RM compared to controls (0.84% vs. 0.37%) has also been reported. Hence, abnormal sperm chromosomes may be associated with RPL. However, at present, there is no test to determine causality of miscarriage due to sperm defects, nor is there any test to determine prognostic significance.

> **PATIENT ADVICE**
>
> Sperm defects may cause RPL, but there is no clinically useful test to determine sperm defects affecting RPL.

Psychological Stress

RPL is always a stressful experience. There are repeated cycles of hope and despair. When women with RM conceive again they exhibit high levels of anxiety, having difficulty getting through each day, general tension, despondence, and premonitions of miscarriage. These feelings may be exhibited by weeping, fear of detecting bleeding, examining underwear, extreme anxiety over any abdominal pain, constant checking continuously for signs of pregnancy, avoidance of other pregnant women, and reluctance to discuss the pregnancy with anyone, including husbands. However, it is unclear whether stress may cause miscarriage. Studies in rodents have suggested that stress increases the rates of implantation and resorption. Exposing pregnant rats or mice to stress can result in lower pregnancy rates, higher embryonic death, more resorptions, and smaller litters. In a later study, women with high stress scores have been found to have higher numbers of tryptase + mast cells, CD8+ T-cells and TNF-α + cells than women with low stress scores. In addition, the authors group have shown NK cell numbers to increase just from the stress of having blood drawn. The relationship between stress and corpus luteal dysfunction has also been reviewed elsewhere.

Prognosis in pregnancy

As stated earlier, the subsequent pregnancy is also accompanied by much stress as the patient remains at a high risk for early and later obstetric complications.

The incidence of vaginal bleeding is found in approximately 40% of pregnancies which develop. The incidence of fetal anomalies is also increased. In late pregnancy, there is an increased incidence of gestational diabetes, pregnancy induced hypertension, intrauterine growth retardation, and preterm labor. Late obstetric complications have been described in APS and hereditary thrombophilias. However, there is insufficient evidence at present to determine whether the late obstetric complications occur exclusively in these two conditions, or whether they are associated with RM per se (see Chapter 11). However, there are prognostic signs in pregnancy which can reassure the patient (and physician). A large number of patients repeatedly lose blighted ova, in whom no heartbeat is ever detected. In these patients, the detection of a fetal heartbeat on ultrasound indicates that the pregnancy is developing differently to previous pregnancies. The likelihood of a pregnancy loss after the detection of fetal heartbeats has been reported as 69/359 (14.2%) in Li *et al*'s series and 22.7% of 185 study patients with multiple spontaneous abortions in different series. If the patient reaches the second trimester with a live fetus, she can also be assured of a good prognosis if she has had previous first trimester abortions.

Classification of prognosis

Brigham *et al*. (1999) have constructed a table to calculate the chance of a subsequent live birth for unexplained RPL, according to the patient's age and number of previous miscarriages. The figures range from a 92% live birth rate for patients age 20 with two miscarriages to 42% for women of age 45 with five miscarriages; however, the 42% live birth rate was based on very few patients and had very wide 95% confidence limits (22–62%). The weakness of Brigham *et al*.'s (1999) study is that it does not include patients with above five miscarriages, and a poorer prognosis. Lund *et al*.'s (2012) study also includes patients with six or more miscarriages, and indicates how many achieve a live birth within a given time span. The author tends to classify patients into those with a good, medium, or poor prognosis (Table 5.2).

Table 5.2 Relative Prognoses According to Clinical Features According to Clinical Features (Carp, 2007)

	Good Prognosis	Medium Prognosis	Poor Prognosis
No. of miscarriages	2 3	4	5 6 7 8 9
Age	20s	30s	40s
Karyotype of abortus	Aberrant	Normal	Normal
1° or 2° Aborter	2°	1° or 3°	1° or 3°
Early or late losses	Early	Early	Late
Infertility	Normal fertility		Infertility
APCA	Positive	Negative	Negative
NK cells	Normal		High

Reprinted from "Recurrent Pregnancy Loss: Causes, Controversies and Treatment" Ed. Carp, HJA. Informa Healthcare, London, UK. 2007. Courtesy of Informa Healthcare.

Good Prognosis

Good prognosis patients are young women with two or possibly three first trimester miscarriages. They probably require little investigation, but do require reassurance of their prognosis, and "tender loving care." Ultrasound scans on a regular basis can reassure the patient and their partner that the pregnancy is progressing normally. The patient should be reassured that in the event of another miscarriage; further investigations will be carried out, including karyotyping of the abortus, and possibly embryoscopy. It is doubtful whether "good prognosis" patients require empirical pharmacological support. A question arises regarding patients who have undergone partial investigations. For example, if a patient with two blighted ova is found to have a septum, it is questionable whether the septum is the cause, or whether should be resected. These questions should be discussed with the patient and partner. In any RM clinic, the majority of patients will have a good prognosis. Their good prognosis should not influence the management of patients with a poor prognosis.

Medium Prognosis Patients

This group of patients will include women with three and possibly four miscarriages. The prognosis for a live birth is approximately 60% after three miscarriages (40% after four miscarriages). We believe that these patients should be investigated. In this group of patients, investigation may vary depending on the clinical presentation. In "medium prognosis" patients, treatment should be directed at the cause as far as possible. However, despite extensive investigations, the cause is often not apparent. In these cases, there may be a place for empirical hormone support with progesterone or hCG, as there is evidence, although debatable, that these hormones may improve the prognosis by approximately 25%. However, treatment is empiric, as there is no investigation in the interval between pregnancies, which can diagnose a hormonal deficiency. A problem may arise when the clinical presentation is at variance with the laboratory investigations. For example, should a patient with aPLs and a chromosomally abnormal abortus in a previous pregnancy be treated by anticoagulants? As with "good prognosis" patients, skill and experience may be necessary to interpret the results.

> **PATIENT ADVICE**
>
> Patients can be classified as good, medium, or poor prognosis depending on the number of miscarriages, age, etc.
> Patients with a good prognosis may not require active treatment.
> Patients with a poor prognosis should be treated, and their therapy should not be deferred due to a good prognosis in "good prognosis patients."

Poor Prognosis Patients

These are the patients with five or more consecutive miscarriages. They have been poorly described in the literature, and have formed the subjects of few trials. The author has previously reported that these patients constitute approximately 20% of the patients in the Recurrent Miscarriage Immunotherapy Trialists Group register, and 30% of the patients in our service. The Sheba Medical Center acts as a tertiary referral center for patients with RPL, which may explain the higher number of patients with a poor prognosis in our service. The feature which distinguishes these patients is that they have usually had all the investigations and empirical treatments available. Hormone supplements, anticoagulants, hysteroscopic surgery, and often in vitro fertilization have been tried. Additionally, there may be APS patients who have failed treatment, patients who continue miscarrying after surgery for uterine anomalies, and in our service, patients who have been treated with anticoagulants for hereditary thrombophilias without success. However, most of these patients have not had fetal karyotyping performed. After five or more miscarriages, the chance of fetal chromosomal aberrations is less than after three miscarriages. Our approach in these patients is to perform alloimmune testing. This will include a cytotoxic cross match between maternal serum and paternal cells to detect APCA. Although the absence of these antibodies may not be relevant after three miscarriages, after five or more miscarriages the absence of these antibodies indicates a poorer prognosis. The numbers and activity of NK cells can also be helpful.

As with the "medium prognosis" patients, we attempt to karyotype the embryo. If immunotherapy fails, and the embryo is karyotypically normal, surrogacy may offer the only possibility of a live birth. If, however, the pregnancy is karyotypically abnormal, a second pregnancy can be attempted with immunotherapy, as immunotherapy cannot prevent chromosomal aberrations. If, however, the patient loses two karyotypically abnormal embryos PGS should be offered, as it is then necessary to ensure that a subsequent pregnancy has a chromosomally normal embryo.

Conclusions

In conclusion, it can be said that RPL is not a homogeneous condition. There is not one prognosis. Various publications in the literature have substantially increased our understanding of the prognosis of RPL. Hopefully, additional information coming available and the introduction of effective treatment regimens will improve the prognosis and move the patients who are now in the poor or medium prognosis group into the good prognosis group.

Bibliography

Brigham, S.A., Conlon, C. and Farquharson, R.G. (1999) A longitudinal study of pregnancy outcome following idiopathic recurrent miscarriage. *Human Reproduction*, **14**, 2868–2871.

Carp, H.J.A. (2007) Investigation protocol for recurrent pregnancy loss, in Recurrent Pregnancy Loss: Causes, Controversies and Treatment (ed H.J.A. Carp), Informa Healthcare, London, pp. 269–280.

Li, T.C., Makris, M., Tomsu, M. et al. (2002) Recurrent miscarriage: aetiology, management and prognosis. Human Reproduction Update, 8, 463–481.

Lund, M., Kamper-Jørgensen, M., Nielsen, H.S. *et al.* (2012) Prognosis for live birth in women with recurrent miscarriage: what is the best measure of success? *Obstetrics and Gynecology*, **119**, 37–43.

Salomon, O., Seligsohn, U., Steinberg, D.M. *et al.* (2004) The common prothrombotic factors in nulliparous women do not compromise blood flow in the feto-maternal circulation and are not associated with preeclampsia or intrauterine growth restriction. *American Journal of Obstetrics and Gynecology*, **191**, 2002–2009.

Sullivan, A.E., Silver, R.M., LaCoursiere, D.Y. *et al.* (2004) Recurrent fetal aneuploidy and recurrent miscarriage. *Obstetrics and Gynecology*, **104**, 784–788.

6

Which Treatments Should be Offered? PGD/PGS, Allogeneic Lymphocyte Immunization, Intravenous Immunoglobulin

Henriette Svarre Nielsen[1] and Ole B. Christiansen[2,3]

[1] Department of Obstetrics and Gynaecology, University of Copenhagen, Copenhagen, Denmark
[2] Unit for Recurrent Miscarriage, Fertility Clinic 4071, Rigshospitalet, Copenhagen, Denmark
[3] Department of Obstetrics and Gynaecology, Aalborg University Hospital, Aalborg, Denmark

Introduction

Relevant and effective treatment options for a disease depend to a large extent on knowledge about the causal mechanisms behind the disease. Recurrent miscarriage (RM) is a unique disease entity as it is defined by a series of events, miscarriages, which, taken individually (sporadic miscarriages), occur in approximately 15% of all pregnancies. Less than 0.5% of women trying to reproduce will by chance experience three sporadic miscarriages (0.15^3) roughly accounting for one third of the RM cases. The remaining two thirds of RM cases are probably associated with (mainly maternal) factors that increase the risk of miscarriage in these couples. The majority of sporadic miscarriages are caused by fetal chromosomal abnormalities incompatible with life. Although the number of chromosomal abnormal miscarriages is found to decrease with increasing number of consecutive miscarriages, all research into effective treatment for RM will be challenged by the high number of miscarriages that are due to chromosomal abnormalities.

RM is a multifactorial disease entity (anatomical, genetic, endocrine, immunological, and vascular) not only at the population level but also within the individual woman, which further challenges the search of effective treatment regimens.

This chapter describes three treatments suggested to improve live birth rates in RM: (i) preimplantation genetic diagnosis (PGD)/preimplantation genetic screening (PGS), (ii) allogeneic lymphocyte immunization, and (iii) intravenous immunoglobulin (IvIg). The theoretical considerations behind each treatment and the studies testing its efficacy will be described.

Recurrent Pregnancy Loss, First Edition. Edited by Ole B. Christiansen.
© 2014 John Wiley & Sons, Ltd. Published 2014 by John Wiley & Sons, Ltd.

Preimplantation genetic testing

Preimplantation genetic testing includes PGD and PGS. The basis for these procedures is in vitro fertilization (IVF). The IVF procedure includes hormone stimulation of the ovaries in order for several eggs to reach the size of maturation and subsequent aspiration. The preimplantation genetic testing can start when the egg is retrieved to test for maternal inherited disease using one or two polar bodies (oocyte nuclei). The other option is to use nuclei from the embryos (blastomeres or trophectoderm) after the oocytes have been fertilized and an embryo has developed. The zona pellucida of the embryo is opened by a sharp glass needle, laser, or acid Tyrode's solution. In the normal procedure, one or two nucleated blastomeres are removed on the third day after fertilization at the 6–8 cell stadium of the embryo. Removal of more than one or two blastomeres potentially has an adverse impact on the development of the embryo. Whether to remove one or two blastomeres depends on the embryo quality and the planned diagnostic procedures. The embryo is then either left in the culture up to the blastocyst stage or cryopreserved until the results of the genetic analysis are known. The whole idea behind these procedures is the final transfer on day 4–5 after oocyte retrieval of healthy embryos to avoid miscarriages, termination of pregnancies as a consequence of later genetic testing (chorion villus biopsies or amniocentesis), or delivery of sick children.

PGD is used to test for a specific mutation or an unbalanced chromosomal rearrangement that is transmitted from a parent carrying a known gene mutation or a balanced chromosomal rearrangement. PGS refers to screening for aneuploidy in embryos of parents known or expected to be chromosomally normal.

Preimplantation Genetic Diagnosis (PGD)

PGD aims to detect a single gene mutation using DNA from the cell nucleus. A vast variety of techniques have over the years been developed to assist PGD.

Polymerase chain reaction (PCR) based assays are used to diagnose monogenic disorders, whereas fluorescence in situ hybridization (FISH) is used to detect structural aberrations. PCR amplifies the relevant segment of the genome containing the gene of interest. Monogenic disorders are often diagnosed indirectly by a classic linkage analysis employing polymorphic microsatellites tightly linked to the gene of interest, and thus usually require prior extended familial analysis. The assay can include a direct analysis of the specific mutation, but polymorphic markers are required to verify the origin of the DNA.

FISH is applied on single intact cells and uses DNA probes labeled with colored fluorochromes that specifically bind to DNA sequences unique to each chromosome. FISH is used to identify translocations, the fusion of two chromosomes (Robertsonian), or exchange of chromosome parts between two different chromosomes (reciprocal translocation). FISH can also be used for identification of aneuploidies like trisomy 21. For inherited sex-chromosome diseases, FISH can be used to determine the sex of the embryo and subsequently avoid transfer of embryos with a disease risk. Examples of the latter are hemophilia and muscular dystrophy.

The short time interval available for analysis and the fact that only one or maximum two cells are available for analysis represent the major challenges related to the use of preimplantation genetic testing. Misdiagnosis can have multiple origins such as failure of amplification of the specific DNA segment, contamination with "foreign" DNA, or contamination with maternal cells during the biopsy procedure. "Allele drop-out" is the result of one allele of the gene under investigation that fails to amplify and partial amplification refers to poor amplification. When testing is performed on a single cell, misdiagnosis may have major consequences: either an affected embryo thought to be normal will be transferred or a nonaffected embryo is discarded. The estimated risk of transferring an affected embryo identified as normal is on average 2% in monogenic disorders but is dependent on the specific kind of analysis. This risk is considered acceptable but prenatal diagnosis, for example, by chorionic villous biopsy is normally recommended.

RM has been directly associated with parental chromosome anomalies, and therefore it has been a standard recommendation to karyotype the couples suffering RM. The rationale of such chromosome testing has been to identify balanced chromosomal rearrangements that potentially lead to fetal unbalanced rearrangement and subsequent miscarriage. This practice has been challenged by two Dutch and a recent British study. The latter was based on data from four UK centers serving a population of 12.2 million and retrospectively looked at a 5–30 years period. A total of 20 432 individuals were karyotyped due to RM and 406 (1.9%) structural balanced abnormalities were detected. During the corresponding period only four unbalanced karyotypes were identified at prenatal diagnosis in subsequent pregnancies among these couples referred due to a balanced rearrangement in a parent ascertained for RM. The authors estimate a price of approximately one million pounds to find one fetus with unbalanced karyotype when the karyotyping is performed due to RM. These findings raise doubts regarding the cost-effectiveness of current recommendation to carry out karyotyping of couples suffering from RM (see Chapter 2).

In addition, detecting an unbalanced parental karyotype is only a partial explanation of the couples' reproductive problems. In one study, in a cohort of 51 carriers of a structural chromosome rearrangement ascertained on the basis of RM, the miscarried embryos were karyotyped and only 36% were found with unbalanced chromosomal abnormalities – this fact obviously limits the efficacy of selecting embryos by PGD in order to decrease miscarriage risk in these couples.

PGD has shown to be a major scientific advance in couples with a heritable genetic disease. Whether PGD improves live birth rate in couples with RM carrying a structural chromosome abnormality is not investigated either in randomized controlled trials or in nonrandomized comparative studies. The impact of PGD in RM couples may be limited based on the low frequency of unbalanced fetal chromosome rearrangements found at prenatal diagnosis and the finding that only one third of the miscarriages in couples carrying structural chromosome rearrangements and suffering RM have unbalanced karyotypes. In this context it is important to remember that discarding of abnormal embryos or embryos with inconclusive results after genetic analysis will reduce the pregnancy rates after IVF with PGD.

A 2011 systematic review looked at the reproductive outcomes after PGD in couples with RM carrying a structural chromosome abnormality. The reproductive outcome reported in four observational studies of 469 couples after natural conception was compared to that of 126 couples after PGD as reported in 21 studies. Direct comparison between PGD and natural conception in RM couples carrying a structural chromosome abnormality was not possible due to the lack of randomized controlled trials. The time required to obtain a healthy live birth or the live birth rate in a fixed time period would be the best measure of comparisons. None of the studies included these data. Due to the heterogeneity of the studies, a meta-analysis was not appropriate to carry out. After natural conception the median live birth rate was 55.5% (ranging from 33–60%) and after PGD 31% (ranging from 0–100%). Based on these data the authors conclude that there are insufficient data indicating that PGD improves live birth rate in couples with RM carrying a structural chromosome abnormality.

Preimplantation Genetic Screening (PGS)

Among couples with RM, PGS is intended to screen for aneuploidies which will result in miscarriages. As for chromosomal investigation by PGD, the standard procedure for PGS is FISH. This procedure is used to identify the copy number of selected chromosomes. Between 9 and 11 chromosome pairs from each cell can be analyzed by FISH, which is a limitation of this screening procedure. Usually the chromosomes that are chosen for evaluation are those involved in the most common aneuploidies identified in miscarriages. Comparative genomic hybridization (CGH) is an alternative method that can test the entire genome. The CGH technique is based on simultaneous amplification of test and reference samples. Red fluorochromes are used for the test sample and green for the reference sample. The products are allowed to hybridize with a normal male metaphase chromosome spread for 2–3 days. The relative amounts of red and green signal are then processed to determine the chromosome numbers and identify any structural chromosome abnormalities. Whole genome analysis can also be performed using newer methods such as gene chips.

The technical limitations related to PGS are obvious as less than half of the 23 chromosome pairs can be evaluated by the FISH method. Studies comparing FISH and CGH have shown that up to 25% of aneuploid embryos are judged normal by FISH because the abnormal chromosome pairs were not among those included in the FISH analysis. CGH would then be the analysis of choice but this method is limited by the time need for analysis, and therefore this procedure requires embryo cryopreservation as it cannot be completed in the short interval between cell biopsy and embryo transfer. Another important limitation of PGS is related to observations that up to half of all embryos identified as aneuploid at the cleavage stage which survive to the blastocyst stage will end up to be chromosomally normal. This has been explained by embryonic mosaicism at the cleavage stage with subsequent reduced proliferative potential of abnormal cell lines, self-correction of the abnormal cell lines, or a false positive or incorrect result of earlier analysis. The conclusion is that an abnormal result obtained by FISH analysis of a single blastomere removed from a day 3 embryo does not necessarily indicate that the embryo is abnormal.

The rationale of using PGS in couples with unexplained RM is that aneuploidy of the embryo may be the cause of the repeated miscarriages. Data from the European Society of Human Reproduction and Embryology show an increased number of PGS treatments offered to couples with RM during the recent years. A systematic review was published in 2011 looking at the pregnancy outcome after PGS or natural conception in couples with unexplained RM. As for PGD no randomized controlled trials or comparative studies were found. As no study compared PGS to natural conception the authors of the review searched for cohort studies or randomized trials where outcome after natural conception was compared with an intervention other than PGS. This search revealed seven studies where the outcome after natural conception in placebo-treated groups (six studies) or expectant management (one study) was reported. Due to the great heterogeneity of the studies, a meta-analysis was not performed but the tabulated data and listing of ranges were presented. Four observational studies including 10–58 couples were found regarding PGS in RM patients. The mean number of previous miscarriages varied between 2.8 and 4.7. The live birth rate after an average of 1.3 PGS cycles was 35% (ranging from 19–46%). In the seven studies on natural conception the mean number of prior miscarriages ranged from 3.0–5.6 and the mean live birth rate per pregnancy after natural conception was 41%. The miscarriage rate for the PGS group was 9%, which may be lower than the 28% in the natural conception group. With the available literature there seems to be no or limited impact using PGS in unexplained RM. However, randomized controlled trials are needed before sound recommendations can be given for the use of PGS in this disorder. Since conception after PGS normally requires more PGS cycles than just 1.3, as reported earlier, conception after PGS is expected to take longer time than natural conception and therefore the most appropriate way to compare pregnancy outcome after PGS versus natural conception is to register live birth rate per time unit, for example, per year in the two groups. This has so far not been done.

⬡ SCIENCE REVISITED

Parental chromosome testing for balanced structural chromosome abnormalities does not seem to be cost-effective in couples with RM as only very few unbalanced abnormalities are present at subsequent prenatal screening.

Only 36% of miscarriages in RM couples with balanced structural chromosome abnormalities are unbalanced, thereby limiting the potential of PGD to reduce risk of miscarriage in these couples.

There are limited data on the efficacy of PGD in RM patients with structural chromosome abnormalities.

Current evidence does not suggest any benefit of PGD in RM patients with structural chromosome abnormalities.

⬡ SCIENCE REVISITED

PGS is in unexplained RM suggested to reduce the risk of miscarriage due to aneuploid embryos.

An abnormal result by PGS does not necessarily indicate that the embryo is abnormal.

There are no controlled or comparative studies on PGS in unexplained RM patients.

Current evidence does not suggest any benefit of PGS in unexplained RM patients.

Active and passive immunization using lymphocyte immunization and IvIg

Numerous studies have attempted to detect immunological abnormalities in RM patients that may cause the repeated maternal rejection of normal fetuses. Unexplained RM has been interpreted as repeated rejections of the fetal semiallograft or being caused by deficient immunological tolerance to fetal or trophoblastic antigens. Treatments proved to be effective in organ transplantation or autoimmune disease and have therefore been investigated in these patients. Suggested immunological abnormalities in RM patients include (i) a change toward a T helper type 1 dominance in RM patients compared to the T helper type 1/T helper type 2 balance in normal pregnancies resulting in a proinflammatory maternal–fetal environment, (ii) defects in molecular immunosuppressive factors (cytokines and growth factors) at the local decidual/trophoblast level, (iii) abnormal levels or activity of systemic or uterine natural killer (NK) cells. Experimental models of miscarriage have focused on the placental milieu, showing that pregnancy survival depends on inhibition of local inflammatory mediators. Complement inhibitory proteins, maternal regulatory T-cells, tryptophan catabolizing enzymes, and immunoregulatory cytokines have been found to allow immunotolerance at the maternal–fetal interface. Cellular and humoral immunological dysfunction in women with unexplained RM may in theory be corrected or modified by various modalities of immune therapy.

Treatment with prednisone generally dampens allo- and autoimmune reactions and will be discussed in Chapter 7 and rarely used therapies with TNF-α inhibitors or G-CSF will be reviewed in Chapter 8. Here we will review the current knowledge regarding two other widely used forms of immunotherapy: active immunization using partner (PLT) or donor lymphocyte therapy (DLT) and passive immunization using IvIg.

Allogeneic Lymphocyte Immunization

Immunological recognition of the pregnancy is critical for the maintenance of gestation. So-called active immunization with lymphocytes from the partner (PLT) or third party donors (DLT) has been widely used within and outside controlled trials since 1980. These treatments have been suggested to improve the immunological recognition by establishing microchimerism, modifying cytokine production, dampening NK cell activity, and producing antipaternal or blocking antibodies.

In 1994, a meta-analysis of all placebo-controlled trials (both PLT and DLT trials) showed that allogeneic lymphocyte transfusion or injection significantly increased the chance of live birth with 16.3% (95% CI 4.8–27.8%) among patients with primary RM (a series of miscarriages with no prior birth(s)) and no auto- or allo-antibodies, whereas no effect could be detected in patients with secondary RM (miscarriages subsequent to a birth). The use of allogeneic lymphocyte administration became a quite widespread and accepted treatment until 1999, at which time the results of a large placebo-controlled trial showed that PLT did not increase the chance of live birth compared with placebo but rather tended to decrease it. This trial has been criticized since the lymphocytes used for transfusions were stored overnight before infusion and because the live birth rate among the immunized patients was much lower than that reported in similar trials. Controversies thus still remain whether allogeneic lymphocyte administration is effective or not. Almost all trials on this therapy have tested PLT, whereas only three trials have tested DLT including a total of 156 patients. The 2006 Cochrane meta-analysis of placebo-controlled trials found that the odds ratio (OR) for live birth after PLT was 1.23 (95% CI 0.89–1.70) and for DLT 1.39 (95% CI 0.68–2.82) and concluded that neither treatment provides significant beneficial effect over placebo in preventing further miscarriages.

This conclusion has been criticized as the therapeutic benefit of PLT, and especially DLT may become statistically significant if more studies were included. As mentioned, the meta-analysis on DLT was based on only three small trials. Also there is evidence that intravenous administration of high doses of an antigen in the absence of additional costimulatory signal (as done on DLT) is a better way to induce tolerance compared to subcutaneous/intradermal administration of smaller doses of an antigen as normally used in PLT. Therefore, there seems to be room for more randomized controlled trials testing DLT using intravenous administration.

In 2006, in a Cochrane review it was stated that the Director of the Office of Therapeutics Research and Review, United States Food and Drug Administration, had sent a letter on January 30, 2002, to physicians believed to be using allogeneic lymphocyte immune therapy to prevent miscarriages. He informed them that the injectable products used in lymphocyte immune therapy do not have the required FDA approval and are considered investigational new drugs that pose several significant safety concerns. Administration of such cells or cellular products in humans can only be performed in the United States as part of clinical investigations, and then only if there is an Investigational New Drug application (IND) in effect. All institutions, reproductive centers, and physicians were reminded that they should not administer allogeneic cells or cellular products to miscarriage patients until an IND has been submitted and reviewed by the FDA's Center for Biologics Evaluation and Research.

Since allogeneic lymphocyte therapy theoretically poses serious side effects such as maternal production of anti-red-cell and platelet antibodies, transmission of viruses and prions, suppression of the immune defense against infections, and maybe an increased risk of certain cancer forms this treatment should as a main rule only be given in the context of randomized controlled trials. However, acknowledging the OR 1.39 for live birth after DLT compared with placebo, the authors of this chapter believe that in a few instances: in patients with PRM and multiple miscarriages in spite of all other treatment, intravenous DLT could be tried if the patients are clearly informed of the limited evidence for effect and possible side effects.

SCIENCE REVISITED

Active allogeneic immunization using third party donor lymphocyte transfusions in primary RM may improve live birth rate based on randomized controlled trials.

Partner lymphocyte transfusion may, according to randomized controlled trials, exhibit a small positive effect on live birth rate in primary RM.

Future studies should focus on immune parameters that may predict pregnancy success when using active lymphocyte immunization.

> **⚠ CAUTION**
>
> Allogeneic lymphocyte therapy may induce production of red-cell and platelet antibodies that may cause later neonatal problems. This risk can be eliminated using lymphocytes from blood donors matching the patients for the most important red-cell and platelet antigens.
>
> Allogeneic lymphocyte therapy may in theory have a long term negative impact of the mothers' immune function, an aspect which must be discussed with the patients before offering the treatment.

Intravenous Immunoglobulin (IvIg)

IvIg is a fractionated blood product prepared from the serum of between 1000 and 15 000 donors per batch. High dose IvIg is used as an immunomodulatory agent in immune and inflammatory disorders. The clinical specialities using the largest amounts of IvIg are neurology, hematology, immunology, nephrology, rheumatology, and dermatology. As an immunological background is suggested for unexplained RM, several trials have tested the efficacy of IvIg to increase live birth rates in this disorder. In 2006–7 two systematic reviews were published pooling the randomized trials testing the effectiveness of IvIg in treating RM; however, they reached different conclusions. IvIg did not improve live birth rate in RM according to Porter *et al.* (2006) in an analysis not making separate analyses in primary and secondary RM. In the other meta-analysis Hutton *et al.* (2007) differentiated between primary and secondary RM and reported IvIg to increase the chance of a live birth in secondary RM (OR 2.71, 95% CI 1.09–6.73) but did not find any evidence for its use in primary RM (OR 0.66, 95% CI 0.35–1.26). Although differentiation seems reasonable the results need to be understood with caution. The evidence of benefit of IvIg for secondary RM was based on four studies. The included trials are heterogenic, have limited number of patients, differ in severity (number of prior miscarriages) and treatment regimen. In some trials, IvIg was only initiated at the time of demonstration of fetal heart action in gestational week 7, whereas in other trials treatment was started at the time of a positive pregnancy test or even before conception. In addition, the doses and the infusion intervals varied significantly between trials. In 2010, a new randomized controlled trial with a total of 47 patients testing IvIg specifically in secondary RM was published. Live birth rate was 70% in the IvIg treatment group and 63% in the placebo group (OR 1.37, 95% CI 0.41–4.61). As part of reporting the last trial, a meta-analysis was combining the results of the trial with two of the prior four trials testing IvIg in secondary RM. When combining the results of these three trials, IvIg did not seem to improve the live birth rate compared to placebo. However, if the two omitted studies were included, IvIg would significantly improve live birth rate. Given these diverse results no clear recommendation can be given at the moment whether or not to treat women with IvIg if suffering secondary RM. The final answer in this discussion will hopefully be provided from the ongoing trial http://clinicaltrials.gov that is almost completed and will include a total of 82 women with secondary RM and four or more miscarriages treated with high doses of IvIg, starting very early in pregnancy.

SCIENCE REVISITED

IvIg is a blood product from pooled plasma from thousands of donors used as an immunomodulatory agent in immune and inflammatory disorders.

A 2006 meta-analysis of randomized controlled trials suggested that IvIg increases the live birth rate in secondary RM patients; however, a 2010 randomized controlled trial did not find a significant benefit of the treatment in this patient subset.

A large randomized controlled trial is almost completed and will hopefully provide the final answer whether to use IvIg in secondary RM.

CAUTION

Miscarriages due to chromosomal abnormalities will dilute any treatment effect by treatments effective for other causes of RM.

Bibliography

Christiansen, O.B., H.S, N. and B, P. (2004) Active or passive immunization in unexplained recurrent miscarriage. *Journal of Reproductive Immunology*, **62** (1-2), 41–52.

Franssen, M.T.M., A M, M., van der Veen, F. *et al.* (2011) Reproductive outcome after PGD in couples with recurrent miscarriage carrying a structural chromosome abnormality: a systematic review. *Human Reproduction Update*, **17** (4), 467–75.

Hutton, B., Sharma, R., Fergusson, D. *et al.* (2007) Use of intravenous immunoglobulin for treatment of recurrent miscarriage: a systematic review. *BJOG*, **114** (2), 134–42.

Musters A. M., Repping, S., Korevaar, J.C. *et al.* (2011) Pregnancy outcome after preimplantation genetic screening or natural conception in couples with unexplained recurrent miscarriage: a systematic review of the best available evidence *Fertility and Sterility* **95** (6): 2153–2157.

Porter TF, LaCoursiere Y, Scott JR. Immunotherapy for recurrent miscarriage. *Cochrane Database Systematic Reviews* 2006; **2**: CD000112.

7

Which Treatment Should be Offered? Heparin/Aspirin, Progesterone, Prednisolone

Muhammad A. Akhtar[1] and Siobhan Quenby[2]

[1] Reproductive Medicine Unit, University Hospitals Coventry and Warwickshire NHS Trust, University of Warwick, Coventry, UK
[2] Reproductive Health, Warwick Medical School, University of Warwick, Coventry, UK

Introduction

Recurrent miscarriage (RM) is very distressful situation for a woman and her family. It has a significant psychological, social, and physical morbidity for women. There are about 12 000 couples a year in England and Wales suffering RMs. Treatment of RMs is very challenging as it is difficult to ascertain the cause or associated factors for each and repeated miscarriages. The only widely accepted treatable cause for RM is antiphospholipid syndrome that affects about 10% of couples. Hence for 90% of couples suffering this condition, there is no accepted treatment.

There are very few good-quality trials done to look for the efficacy of treatments for RM. The current data from four published Cochrane reviews regarding RM shows a total number of women involved in trials of sufficient quality to be included in the Cochrane review of trials to be a total of 4000 worldwide over 50 years. The Cochrane review currently recommends that there is insufficient evidence to justify the treatments in RM and all need further investigation. This is because insufficient improvements in live birth rates in subsequent pregnancies have been found in meta-analyses of RCTs of treatment. However, all women can be offered supportive care in subsequent pregnancies since the live birth rates with this in the control/placebo arm of RCTs have been high (60–80%).

In order to rectify this situation, several large-scale RCTs are being conducted currently. An example of these is the PROMISE trial of progesterone against placebo for idiopathic RM. The power calculation indicated that this requires 790 women to be randomized in order to substantiate any benefit for progesterone supplementation. There has never been published a trial of this size in RM research.

Recurrent Pregnancy Loss, First Edition. Edited by Ole B. Christiansen.
© 2014 John Wiley & Sons, Ltd. Published 2014 by John Wiley & Sons, Ltd.

The current situation of a lack of evidence leads to widespread use of empirical treatment in idiopathic RM. A better option may be to encourage women to participate in high-quality and methodologically sound studies to guide optimal management.

Heparin and aspirin

Low doses of aspirin reduce both pain and fever, whereas the anti-inflammatory action of aspirin requires a much higher dose. It is possible that inhibition of cyclooxygenase (COX)-1 is the major action of aspirin involved in its analgesic and antipyretic effects, and inhibition of COX-2 is responsible for its anti-inflammatory action. Aspirin has an antiplatelet effect, so it is used long-term, at low doses, to help prevent heart attacks, stroke, and blood clot formation.

> ### ⬡ SCIENCE REVISITED
>
> Low-dose acetylsalicylic acid (aspirin) irreversibly inhibits the enzyme cyclooxygenase in platelets, preventing the synthesis of thromboxane. The daily administration of aspirin in low doses induces a shift in the balance away from thromboxane A2 and toward prostacyclin, leading to vasodilatation and increased blood perfusion.

Heparin is effective for the prevention and treatment of venous thrombosis and pulmonary embolism. Traditionally, the role of heparin is prevention of thrombosis in relation to implantation and placental development for women with inherited and acquired thrombophilia. But there is a potential role for heparin in assisted conception due to its ability to interact with a wide variety of proteins, for example, selectins, cadherins, heparin-binding epidermal growth factor, insulin-like growth factor (IGF-I and IGF-II), which can alter the physiological processes of implantation and trophoblast development. Heparin is also protective against trophoblast apoptosis.

> ### ⬡ SCIENCE REVISITED
>
> Heparin is a sulfated polysaccharide with a molecular weight range of 3000–30 000 Da (mean, 15 000 Da). It produces its major anticoagulant effect by inactivating thrombin and activated factor X (factor Xa) through an antithrombin (AT)-dependent mechanism.
>
> Low-molecular-weight Heparin (LMWH) is derived from heparin by enzymatic (e.g., tinzaparin) or chemical (e.g., dalteparin, nadroparin, and enoxaparin) depolymerization of unfractionated heparin (UFH), which in itself cannot be synthesized in vitro.

> ### ⬡ SCIENCE REVISITED
>
> **Early Pregnancy Development**
>
> In normally developing pregnancies, intervillous blood flow starts only between 8 and 12 weeks of gestation and is consistently present only from 12 weeks of

gestation. Hence, the end of the first trimester is characterized by a progressive increase in blood flow, oxygenation, and oxidative stress. First trimester miscarriage has been characterized by early and excessive placental blood flow. Thus, in this biological framework, it is unlikely that thrombosis leading to a reduction in blood loss is a contributory factor in early miscarriage and that prevention of thrombosis will prevent early miscarriage.

Clinical data

Clinical thinking about aspirin and heparin for the prevention of miscarriage has been highly influenced by the Cochrane review "Prevention of recurrent miscarriage for women **with** antiphospholipid antibody or lupus anticoagulant." This concluded that: "Combined unfractionated heparin and aspirin may reduce pregnancy loss by 54%. Large RCTs with adequate allocation concealment are needed to explore potential differences between unfractionated heparin and LMWH."

This finding of a potential 54% reduction in pregnancy loss lead to the clinical interpretation that thromboprophylaxis was beneficial to early pregnancy.

In 2009, the Cochrane published a review "Aspirin or anticoagulants for treating recurrent miscarriage in women without antiphospholipid syndrome" that included two studies (189 participants). Similar live birth rates were observed with aspirin and placebo, both 81% (risk ratio (RR) 1.00, 95% confidence interval (CI) 0.78–1.29), and enoxaparin and aspirin, respectively, 82% and 84% (RR 0.97, 95% CI 0.81–1.16). They concluded that

- There is paucity in studies on the efficacy and safety of aspirin and heparin in women with a history of at least two miscarriages without apparent causes other than inherited thrombophilia.
- The two reviewed trials studied different treatments and only one study was placebo-controlled. Neither of the studies showed a benefit of one treatment over the other.
- The use of anticoagulants in this setting is not recommended.
- Large randomized, placebo-controlled trials are urgently needed.

✋ CAUTION

A key issue for clinical studies is that most studies include losses up to 20 weeks of gestation, although the definition of fetal loss varies. This means that studies may contain women with losses attributable to two different mechanisms. Before 10–12 weeks of gestation, there is no intervillous blood flow; until then, respiration and nutrition are by passive transfer across tissues. Some might argue that such distinctions ignore the reality that embryo–fetal development is truly a continuum. However, contrary to the continuum paradigm, there are clear milestones in development, and the 10–12 week mark is one of these. Thus, "thrombosis of the placenta" as a cause of fetal loss can be ascribed only to losses after the initiation of blood flow at 10–12 weeks of gestation.

Four recent RCTs (HEPSA, HABENOX, SPIN, ALIFE) including women with two or more pregnancy losses have failed to demonstrate any improvement in pregnancy outcome in women with idiopathic RMs with low-dose aspirin with or without LMWH.

The trials were underpowered to confirm or refute an effect in women with three or more losses or those with thrombophilia, although in all trials post hoc subgroup analyses for these factors showed no trend in terms of benefit. These findings are important, as they indicate that the empirical administration of heparin and aspirin in RM should discontinue.

The only place for heparin and aspirin in the prevention of miscarriage in the absence of antiphospholipid antibodies is in well-conducted RCTs of high-risk women. However, in the case of antiphospholipid antibodies and RM, aspirin and heparin are still recommended.

Inherited thrombophilias have been associated with RM, although the prevalences in the general and RM populations vary hugely. There is a lack of pregnancy outcome data with individual coagulation abnormalities and as a result, treatment varies widely. In women with previous thromboembolic disease, LMWH is often used in pregnancy to prevent maternal thrombosis. In women who have had a previous miscarriage, aspirin and LMWH are increasingly used with the aim of preventing both miscarriage and maternal thrombosis.

- The HepASA trial recruited women with a history of two or more miscarriages and at least one of the following: antiphospholipid antibody, an inherited thrombophilia, and/or antinuclear antibody. Out of the 859 women who were screened, 88 became pregnant and were randomized to receive low-dose aspirin and LMWH (dalteparin) or low-dose aspirin alone. There were no differences in the live birth rate between the two groups (77.8 vs. 79.1%).
- The SPIN, ALIFE, and HABENOX trials also included women with or without inherited or acquired thrombophilias, and the subset analyses of these found no benefit from either low-dose aspirin or low-dose aspirin and LMWH above absence of pharmaceutical treatment in these women.

Moreover, as the majority of trials of RMs contain women with miscarriages before 12 weeks of gestation, the effect of heparin and aspirin is not being properly assessed in those with losses after 12 weeks of gestation; that is, in the second trimester. There are suggestions (evidence cannot be obtained from pilot studies) from two pilot trials of LMWH that the use of antithrombotics may be effective in preventing placental thrombosis after 12 weeks of gestation. In support of the concept of a gestation-specific effect of antithrombotic treatment on miscarriage risk is the finding that low-dose aspirin has a moderate effect at preventing preeclampsia in the second and third trimesters.

Progesterone

Scientific Rational

Progesterone is known to induce secretory changes and decidual differentiation in the endometrium of the uterus essential for successful implantation of a fertilized egg.

It suppresses myometrial contractility. It maintains corpus luteum function longer for maintenance of pregnancy.

Clinical Data

Fifteen trials (2118 women) are included in the Cochrane review "progestogens for preventing miscarriage." The meta-analysis of all women, regardless of gravidity and number of previous miscarriages, showed no statistically significant difference in the risk of miscarriage between progestogen and placebo or no treatment groups (Peto odds ratio (Peto OR) 0.98; 95% CI 0.78–1.24) and no statistically significant difference in the incidence of adverse effect in either mother or baby. In a subgroup analysis of three trials involving women who had RMs (three or more consecutive miscarriages), progestogen treatment showed a statistically significant decrease in miscarriage rate compared to placebo or no treatment (Peto OR 0.38; 95% CI 0.20–0.70). No statistically significant differences were found between the route of administration of progestogen (oral, intramuscular, vaginal) versus placebo or no treatment.

⚗ SCIENCE REVISITED

It has been suggested that a causative factor in many cases of miscarriage may be inadequate secretion of progesterone during the luteal phase of the menstrual cycle and in the early weeks of pregnancy. Therefore, progestogens have been used, beginning in the first trimester of pregnancy, in an attempt to prevent miscarriage. However, whilst low progesterone levels in early pregnancy undoubtedly predict failure, these low levels could be the result rather than the cause of the failing pregnancy.

The authors concluded that there is no evidence to support the routine use of progestogen to prevent miscarriage in early to mid-pregnancy. However, there seems to be evidence of benefit in women with a history of RM. Treatment for these women may be warranted given the reduced rates of miscarriage in the treatment group and the finding of no statistically significant difference between treatment and control groups in rates of adverse effects suffered by either mother or baby in the available evidence. Larger trials (PROMISE) are currently underway to provide information about the treatment for this group of women.

Future research

This randomized, double-blind, placebo-controlled multicenter trial (PROMISE) is studying the effect of progesterone treatment given in the first trimester of pregnancy in women with a history of unexplained RMs. The total number of participants required will be **790** (395 in each trial arm) to detect a minimally important difference of 10% in live birth beyond 24 weeks (from 60% to 70%) for an alpha error rate of 5% and beta error rate of 20%, after adjustment for a loss to follow-up rate of 5%.

> **✋ CAUTION**
>
> Concerns have been raised that the use of progestogens, with their uterine-relaxant properties, in women with fertilized defective ova may cause a delay in miscarriage.
>
> Several reports also suggest an association between intrauterine exposure to progesterone containing drugs in the first trimester of pregnancy and genital abnormalities in male and female fetuses. The risk of hypospadias (deformities of the penis or urethra, or both), 5–8 per 1000 male births in the general population, may be approximately doubled with exposure to these drugs. There are insufficient data to quantify the risk to exposed female fetuses, but due to some reports stating these drugs induce mild virilization (masculinization) of the external genitalia of the female fetus, and because of the increased association of hypospadias in the male fetus, it has been recommended that progesterone-containing drugs be avoided in the first 3 months of pregnancy. However, the meta-analysis showed no statistically significant difference in the number of fetal abnormalities (including virilization and hypospadias) in babies whose mothers had been given progestogens whilst in vitro or in intrauterine death/still birth or neonatal death.

Prednisolone

- Scientific rational

Prednisolone is a corticosteroid drug with predominant glucocorticoid and low mineralocorticoid activity, Prednisolone irreversibly binds with glucocorticoid receptors (GR) alpha and beta for which they have a high affinity.

> **♺ SCIENCE REVISITED**
>
> Uterine Natural Killer (uNK) cells are characterized by the presence of CD56 antigen and the absence of the CD16 and CD4 antigens. Thus uNK cells are different from the majority of peripheral NK cells that express both CD56 and CD16. uNK cells are, numerically, the most important leucocytes in preimplantation endometrium and early pregnancy decidua, are maximal in number in the midluteal phase when implantation occurs, and are found adjacent to the fetal extravillous trophoblast in early pregnancy. Furthermore, uNK cells express families of receptors that are capable of recognizing specific antigens on the surface of extravillous trophoblast. Studies on preimplantation endometrium have found increased numbers of uNK cells in women suffering idiopathic RM. Furthermore, high numbers of uNK cells in women with RM predicted miscarriage in subsequent pregnancy. Glucocorticoid receptors have been demonstrated on the surface of uNK.

More recent publications have focused on the role of decidual stromal cells in the maternofetal interaction and the subsequent maintenance of early pregnancy.

Stromal cell expression of the serum- and glucocorticoid-inducible kinase SGK1 expression was lower in RM patients, not only when compared to infertile patients but also to fertile controls. SGK1, a serine/threonine protein kinase homologous to AKT, is rapidly induced in response to a rise in progesterone levels in both human and murine endometrium, first in epithelial cells and then in the decidualizing stroma. SGK1 is a key regulator of sodium transport in mammalian epithelia, most prominently through its ability to directly activate epithelial sodium channels (ENaC) and to enhance their expression by inhibiting the ubiquitin ligase Nedd4-2. SGK1 is also involved in proliferation and cell survival response. In pregnancy, endometrial SGK1 activity safeguards the decidual–placental interface against oxidative stress signals generated in response to the intense tissue remodeling, influx of inflammatory cells, and dynamic changes in local perfusion and oxygen tension. Hence, any increase in SGK1 induced by prednisolone should maintain early pregnancy.

- Clinical data

Prednisolone was demonstrated to reduce high density of uNK cells in preimplantation endometrium of women with RM.

A pilot, double-blind, placebo-controlled, RCT of prednisolone (n = 160) found that it was feasible to recruit women with idiopathic RM into a "screen and treat" trial. There was a trend toward an increased live birth rate with prednisolone therapy (live birth rate of 60% vs. 40%, relative risk 1.5; 95% CI 0.8–2.9; absolute risk difference 20%; 95% CI 11%–48%) in women with abnormal levels of uNK cells. Prednisolone treatment was associated with minimal side effects and there were no significant adverse pregnancy complications for both mother and baby. A larger, definitive trial of 214 women and in excess of 850 endometrial biopsies is needed to confirm or refute these findings.

Side Effects of Prednisolone

Abdominal pain, nausea, headaches, increased appetite, dizziness, oral thrush, mood changes, changes in thoughts and behavior, sleeping difficulties, confusion, blurred vision, muscle weakness, and changes in the menstrual cycle in women.

It also causes increase in blood sugar level and long-term use could cause osteoporosis, glaucoma, and cataract.

Other treatment options

These include bed rest, vitamin supplementation, and early scanning in subsequent pregnancies. There is no evidence available to support that these interventions improve implantation and pregnancy rates after unexplained RMs. However, psychological support in early pregnancy may help improve the outcome.

Estrogen

This should not be used for the treatment of RMs as exposure to diethylstilboestrol in utero increases primary infertility and vaginal adenosis among female offspring and testicular abnormalities in male offspring. It also increases the risk of genital tract cancer.

Conclusion

RMs cause pronounced psychological responses including anxiety, depression, denial, and anger. Careful individual counselling with dignity is required to provide the couple support needed for future.

The treatment of couples with RM has traditionally been based on anecdotal evidence, personal bias, and willingness to help the distressed couple. When assessing the efficacy of any intervention, it is pivotal to recognize that at least one third of couples with a history of three consecutive miscarriages have lost pregnancies purely by chance alone, secondary to sporadic fetal aneuploidy. Such couples have a 75% chance of a successful pregnancy next time with no therapeutic intervention.

At the current time, there is a need for further RCTs of treatment for the prevention of miscarriage in women with RM. Hence, best clinical practice at the moment involved entry into well-designed trials.

Bibliography

Coomarasamy, A. and Rai, R. (2011) Does first trimester progesterone prophylaxis increase the live birth rate in women with unexplained recurrent miscarriages? PROMISE study. *BMJ*, **342**, d1914

Clark, P., Walker, I.D. and Langhorne, P. *et al.* (2010) Scottish Pregnancy Intervention Study (SPIN) Collaborators. SPIN (Scottish Pregnancy Intervention) study: a multicenter randomized controlled trial of low-molecular-weight heparin and low dose aspirin in women with recurrent miscarriage. *Blood*, **115**, 4162–4167.

Empson, M.B., Lassere, M., Craig, J.C, and Scott, J.R. (2005) Prevention of recurrent miscarriage for women with antiphospholipid antibody or lupus anticoagulant. *Cochrane Database of Systematic Reviews* **2** (Art. No.: CD002859), updated September 2005.

Haas D.M. and Ramsey P.S. (2008) Progestogen for preventing miscarriage *Cochrane Database of Systematic Reviews* **2** (Art. NO.: CD003511).

Kaandorp S., Di Nisio M, Goddijn M, and Aspirin or anticoagulants for treating recurrent miscarriage in women without antiphospholipid syndrome. *Cochrane Database of Systematic Reviews* 1 (Art. No.: CD004734).

Kaandorp, S.P., Goddijn, M. and van der Post, J.A. *et al.* (2010) Aspirin plus heparin or aspirin alone in women with recurrent miscarriage. *The New England Journal of Medicine*, **362**, 1586–1596.

Laskin, C.A., Spitzer, K.A. and Clark, C.A. *et al.* (2009) Low molecular weight heparin and aspirin for recurrent pregnancy loss: results from the randomized, controlled HepASA trial. *Journal of Rheumatology*, **36**, 279–287.

Quenby, S.M., Hunt, B.J and Maybury, H.J (June, 2011) The Use of Antithrombotics in the Prevention of Recurrent Miscarriage. Royal College of Obstetricians and Gynaecologists, UK, Scientific Advisory Opinion Paper No 26,

Salker, M.S., Christian, M. and Steel, J.H. *et al.* (2011) Deregulation of the serum- and glucocorticoid-inducible kinase SGK1 in the endometrium causes reproductive failure. *Nature Medicine*, **17** (11), 1509–1513.

Tang A., Alfirevic Z. and Turner M A. *et al.* 2009 Prednisolone trial: study protocol for a randomized controlled trial of prednisolone for women with idiopathic recurrent miscarriage and raised levels of uterine natural killer (uNK) cells in the endometrium. *Trials*, **10**:102

Visser, J., Ulander, V.M. and Helmerhorst, F.M. *et al.* (2011) Thromboprophylaxis for recurrent miscarriage in women with or without thrombophilia. HABENOX: a randomised multicentre trial. *Thrombosis and Haemostasis*, **105**, 205–301.

8

Which Treatment Should be Offered: Metformin, hCG, GM-CSF/G-CSF, TNF-α Inhibitors, Standard IVF/ICSI

Ole B. Christiansen[1,2]

[1] Unit for Recurrent Miscarriage, Fertility Clinic 4071, Rigshospitalet, Copenhagen, Denmark
[2] Department of Obstetrics and Gynaecology, Aalborg University Hospital, Aalborg, Denmark

Introduction

From a strict point of view, all treatments for RM should be considered experimental. Even the use of the most established treatment: heparin and low-dose aspirin in patients with antiphospholipid antibodies is based on three small nonblinded trials with no placebo arm and with large heterogeneity between trials (see Chapter 7).

However, whereas treatments such as heparin, intravenous immunoglobulin, prednisone and allogeneic lymphocyte injections each have been tested in several trials of varying quality (Chapters 6 and 7), some treatments such as administration of metformin, hCG, TNF-α inhibitors, GM-CSF, G-CSF, or the use of IVF/ICSI without preimplantation genetic testing have only been tested in one or two trials in RM patients or tested in women with no history of RM. They must therefore be considered truly experimental.

Since the initial trials of these treatments were very promising or the treatments from a theoretical point of view display a large potential for being efficient, a state-of-the-art review of these treatments is provided.

Metformin

PCOS characterized by oligomenorrhea or amenorrhea, clinical and/or biochemical signs of hyperandrogenism and polycystic appearance of the ovaries by ultrasound has long been suggested to predispose to miscarriage, RM, and late pregnancy complications.

Some studies have found a higher prevalence of PCOS in RM women than in fertile controls, but whether there is any causal association is still controversial. In a large study of women undergoing infertility treatment, the risk of future miscarriage was significantly higher in patients with PCOS compared with those without (25% vs. 18%), but after adjusting for obesity and kind of fertility treatment in a multivariate analysis, the risk of miscarriage became similar in the two groups. The miscarriage rate of 18% in PCOS women was similar to the 19% miscarriage rate found in clomiphene (clomid)-treated PCOS patients in two other large prospective studies. It is generally suggested that the rate of clinical miscarriage per pregnancy in the background population is 12–15%, so the risk in PCOS patients may be slightly higher. One factor that has most consistently been associated with the clinical symptoms of PCOS, including the infertility problems, is hyperandrogenism. Increased levels of androgens can often be detected in blood samples in PCOS patients but even in case of normal plasma levels, intraovarian testosterone production is suggested to be elevated. Hyperinsulinemia is often found in obese individuals and women with PCOS and is suggested to stimulate testosterone production in the ovaries.

Metformin is an insulin-sensitizing drug that suppresses insulin levels in nonpregnant individuals and suppresses androgen levels both in PCOS women with hyperinsulinemia but surprisingly also in women with normal plasma insulin. If elevated androgens (or other factors upregulated by hyperinsulinemia) play a role in infertility, increased miscarriage rate, and late pregnancy complications found in PCOS patients, metformin treatment is expected to be beneficial. A series of trials have therefore tested metformin in PCOS patients with infertility with or without a history of miscarriage. In seven studies, either retrospective or comparing miscarriage rates in the same patients before and after metformin treatment, a statistically significantly lower miscarriage rate was reported in PCOS patients treated with metformin during pregnancy compared with nonmetformin-treated patients. The miscarriage rates in the metformin-treated patients were between 8.8% and 26.1%, which on average may be slightly lower than the previously mentioned 18–19% rate after clomiphene citrate or ART treatment of PCOS patients. However, nonprospective, nonrandomized studies are subject to selection bias and therefore the results from these studies must be interpreted with care.

In contrast, in high-quality, prospective, RCTs where metformin treatment was provided to PCOS patients before conception but halted at the time of positive pregnancy test, the rate of subsequent miscarriage was not decreased compared with patients only treated with clomiphene citrate. Indeed, a recent Cochrane analysis on the topic found that the miscarriage rate in pregnancies conceived during metformin/clomiphene citrate treatment was almost significantly elevated compared to pregnancies conceived by clomiphene citrate treatment alone (OR = 1.61; 95% CI 1.00–2.60).

Furthermore, a recent, large, multicenter RCT did not find that metformin treatment during pregnancy reduced the risk of a series of late pregnancy complications in PCOS patients.

In conclusion, there is no documentation that metformin treatment neither before nor during pregnancy reduces the risk of subsequent miscarriage in PCOS patients with infertility problems. The data concerning RM patients with PCOS are too limited to draw any conclusions whether metformin displays any beneficial effect in this patient subset and there is a need for RCTs to clarify the issue.

⚙ SCIENCE REVISITED

PCOS is weakly associated with an increased risk of miscarriage.

It is unclear whether the increased miscarriage rate is primarily associated with obesity, the treatments offered to the patients, or measurable endocrine disturbances

Metformin has been proven to suppress insulin and androgen levels, which are often elevated in PCOS patients

Metformin treatment until the time of positive pregnancy test does not decrease and may rather increase the miscarriage rate in PCOS patients undergoing fertility treatment

The quality of the studies that have evaluated the effect of metformin treatment during pregnancy in PCOS patients are of limited quality and does not allow any conclusions regarding effects on miscarriage risks

---

hCG

Human chorionic gonadotrophin (hCG) is a glycoprotein composed of two subunits α and β where the α subunit is similar to the α subunit of the gonadotrophins FSH and LH while the β subunit is unique for hCG. Increasing amounts of hCG are secreted by the syncytiotrophoblast with increased gestation in the first trimester and can be measured in plasma from a few days after embryo implantation. Plasma-hCG will normally bind to the LH/hCG receptor on the corpus luteum, preventing it to undergo regression 14 days after ovulation and will stimulate its production of hormones such as estrogen and progesterone that are necessary for early pregnancy survival. After gestational week 7, the progesterone production shifts from the corpus luteum to the placenta, where it is probably independent of plasma-hCG levels.

Early miscarriage is normally associated with low plasma-hCG levels or a sub-normal plasma-hCG increment in addition to low plasma progesterone levels. This association between low hCG production and early miscarriage can be interpreted in two different ways, which may both be correct: (i) low plasma-hCG or inadequately increasing hCG indicate that the trophoblast growth is delayed by various reasons that are unrelated to endocrine disturbances (e.g., embryonal aneuploidy) or (ii) low hCG secretion from an otherwise healthy feto-placental unit may result in inadequate progesterone secretion from the corpus luteum (luteal insufficiency). Whereas the first condition in theory cannot be improved by hCG supplementation, the second condition may be treated by external administration of hCG or progesterone.

hCG supplementation during early pregnancy is therefore a potentially efficient treatment of patients with RM and has thus so far been tested in four RCTs, two of which were, however, small. The data of the trials have been summarized in a Cochrane review, finding that the pooled odds ratio for miscarriage in the hCG-treated patients was 0.26 (95% CI 0.14–0.52) compared with non-hCG-treated controls and the immediate conclusion would be that hCG supplementation is beneficial in RM. However, there was significant heterogeneity between the individual trials. The two earliest trials had severe methodological flaws: none of the trials gave details of the randomization procedures and one trial did not use placebo in the control group. The two trials of better quality only found a nonsignificant trend for a beneficial effect of hCG supplementation. The largest of the trials found a significant effect of hCG supplementation in RM patients with oligomenorrhea, whereas no effect at all could be found in patients with regular cycles.

In conclusion, administration of hCG to RM patients cannot be recommended based on results of the RCTs published so far, primarily due to their limited quality. Since all trials conducted until now point toward an effect of the hCG supplementation, there is an urgent need for new high-quality RCTs testing the treatment. These trials may primarily target patients with oligomenorrhea as suggested in one previous RCT.

⚙ SCIENCE REVISITED

Although a meta-analysis of controlled trials of hCG supplementation for RM suggests that the treatment is beneficial, the quality of the trials is generally too low to recommend use of the treatment.

New high-quality trials on the topic are urgently needed.

New trials may focus on subsets of RM patients such as those with oligomenorrhea.

GM-CSF/G-CSF

GM-CSF and G-CSF are so-called hematopoietic cytokines that stimulates neutrophilic granulocyte proliferation and differentiation and are routinely used in the treatment of neutropenia during cancer chemotherapy and for pretreatment of stem cells donors. GM-CSF has been shown to display a key role in the development and viability of murine and human embryos in vitro and embryonal exposure to GM-CSF is essential for normal trophoblast differentiation and fetal growth and gene programming. In vitro exposure of human embryos to GM-CSF doubles the chance of reaching the blastocyst stadium. Genetically modified mice lacking GM-CSF exhibit an increased rate of fetal loss that can be reversed by exogenous administration of GM-CSF.

One single study has reported that plasma levels of GM-CSF during pregnancy were much lower in women with RM compared to normal pregnancy controls.

G-CSF has been demonstrated to be produced by decidual cells and its receptor c-fms is expressed on trophoblast cells and it has been shown to display a positive effect on trophoblast growth and to decrease embryo resorptions in murine pregnancies.

There is thus plenty of evidence that GM-CSF and G-CSF play a role for early pregnancy survival and it is an obvious thought to test administration of GM-CSF and G-CSF to women with unexplained RM or their in vitro embryos. A recently concluded RCT found that transfer of embryos from women with one or more previous miscarriages grown in IVF culture media supplemented with GM-CSF resulted in pregnancies that miscarried significantly less often than transfer of embryos grown in standard media. Concerning the use of G-CSF, one RCT has been undertaken so far. In this trial, patients with a least four unexplained miscarriages who had previously miscarried in spite of intravenous immunoglobulin (IvIg) treatment were randomized to daily subcutaneous injections with G-CSF or placebo from the sixth day after ovulation to the end of ninth gestational week if they became pregnant. In the G-CSF group, 82.8% of 29 women delivered a healthy child compared with only 48.5% (16/33) in the placebo group ($p < 0.01$). There were no pregnancy complications or malformations in any of the children born after G-CSF.

In addition to this RCT, in a retrospective cohort study, G-CSF treatment was given to 49 patients with repeated miscarriages undergoing IVF/ICSI treatment. The study reported a significantly ($p < 0.05$) higher live birth rate of 32% in patients treated with G-CSF compared with 14% and 13% in controls receiving other medication or no medication, respectively.

No serious side effects in women and children have been reported in these studies but since both GM-CSF and G-CSF are potent hematopoietic drugs, the theoretical possibility of development of hematological disorders in the children will be of concern.

In conclusion, from a theoretical point of view, GM-CSF and G-CSF used in IVF media or administered parentally may be efficient treatment options for women with unexplained RM. However, future recommendations cannot be based on only two RCTs, so more well-designed RCTs are awaited before these treatments can be recommended. It is also important that long-term follow-up of the children born after this therapy confirms that the treatment is not associated with an increased incidence of hematological disease.

> ✋ **CAUTION**
>
> Almost all trials of metformin to PCOS patients and the study of culturing embryos in GM-CSF-containing IVF medium have been undertaken in women with no history of RM and the results can therefore not be directly translated to this patient group

TNF-α inhibitors

Many autoimmune diseases are characterized by increased inflammatory reactions, which in many cases play an important role in the pathogenesis of the diseases. TNF-α is an important proinflammatory cytokine that plays a crucial role in the pathogenic processes of rheumatoid arthritis and Crohn's disease. TNF-α activity can be blocked with monoclonal antibodies against the TNF-α molecule (adalimumab) or against soluble TNF-α receptors (etanercept), which are effective treatments in rheumatoid arthritis. Dominance of T-helper type 1 cytokines and among them TNF-α has repeatedly been suggested to characterize pathological pregnancy outcomes, including RM. Several studies carried out in RM patients have reported that increased plasma levels of TNF-α or high production of TNF-α from peripheral blood lymphocytes during pregnancy are associated with a high frequency of miscarriage or miscarriage of chromosomally normal fetuses. Knowing the proven effect of TNF-α inhibitors in autoimmune diseases and the possible harmful effect of elevated TNF-α production in RM, treatment of RM with TNF-α inhibitors appears an interesting option.

However, treatment with TNF-α inhibitors has so far only been tested in one trial with a control group. In a retrospective study, patients with RM were offered three different treatments: 21 patients received anticoagulation therapy (AC) with low-dose heparin and aspirin, 37 patients received in addition to AC IvIg before and in early pregnancy, and 17 patients received a combination of AC, IvIg, and TNF-α inhibitors. TNF-α inhibitors were administered as 40 mg adalimumab subcutaneously every week or second week or 25 mg etanercept every 84 h starting in the beginning of the conception cycle and continuing to the demonstration of fetal heart action by ultrasound. The subsequent live birth rates were 19% in the AC only group, 54% in the AC + IvIg group, and 71% in the group receiving combined AC + IvIg + TNF-α inhibitor. The live birth rate in the latter group was significantly higher than that of the AC only group ($p < 0.003$). Although these results may indicate a beneficial effect of therapy with TNF-α inhibitors in RM, results from this single study must be interpreted with great care. The allocation to the three treatment groups was partly by the patients' self-selection (much dependent on their economical ability) and partly due to their reproductive history and findings in blood samples. Patients with high peripheral blood natural killer cell cytotoxicity or high frequency of CD56 positive cells were offered IvIg if they could afford it and those with a high TNF-α/IL-10 ratio were offered treatment with TNF-α inhibitors. Due to the many methodological limitations in this study, other clinical trials testing this treatment option are needed. It is clear that a valid testing of TNF-α inhibitors in RM can only be done in prospective RCTs with random and blinded allocation to the different groups. Such a trial may be restricted to patients with documented high TNF-α plasma levels during pregnancy.

🔎 SCIENCE REVISITED

In vitro and animal experiments suggest a role of GM-CSF and G-CSF in embryo development and early fetal and trophoblast development.

High plasma TNF-α levels or high TNF-α production by lymphocytes seem to characterize women with RM and seem to be associated with a decreased pregnancy prognosis.

Prospective clinical trials and retrospective studies in humans have provided preliminary evidence that treating IVF embryos with GM-CSF or women with RM with G-CSF or TNF-α inhibitors decrease the risk of miscarriage, but more trials are needed.

IVF/ICSI without PGD

The potential for implantation after uterine transfer of IVF/ICSI cleavage-stage embryos cultured for 2–3 days after fertilization can be assessed by embryo scoring systems based on the number and size of the blastomers and the granularity of the cytoplasma. Some fertility doctors and many RM patients therefore draw the conclusion that since this scoring system can select between embryos with a good and bad implantation potential, it may also be useful for selecting embryos with a less risk for being miscarried. Some fertility clinics are therefore offering standard IVF/ICSI to RM patients with no conception problems based on the belief that it can improve their prognosis for live birth by selecting of cleavage-stage embryos according to standard methods or by culturing the embryos to the blastocyst stage if possible. However, there are no studies that have investigated the potential of standard IVF/ICSI to decrease the risk of miscarriage in RM patients without conception problems. Indeed many studies have shown that the IVF/ICSI procedure is associated with a higher risk of miscarriage than natural conceived pregnancies (see Chapter 12), so IVF/ICSI to this patient group may in theory worsen the prognosis.

In my view, there are two indications for offering standard IVF/ICSI to RM patients. The first indication is prolonged time to pregnancy after a series of miscarriages. Women in developed countries often try for their first child at an age of 30 years and if they subsequently experience four to five miscarriages, they often end up being in the late 30s. This increased age may partly explain that the interval between conceptions typically increases with increased gravidity in RM patients and this is a cause of concern for the patients feeling that they have now two enemies to fight: the high risk of miscarriage and subfertility. The increasing interpregnancy intervals can be related to the age-related diminished ovarian reserve and egg quality, but can also be related to subtotal tubal damage: at each miscarriage, whether treated conservatively or by medical or surgical methods, there is a risk of tubal infection that can damage the tubes. Patients with RM and prolonged time to pregnancy should be offered intrauterine insemination after having failed to conceive after 6 months and if they do not conceive or only experience a biochemical pregnancy after insemination, they should immediately continue with IVF/ICSI. They should be clearly told that IVF/ICSI treatment during these circumstances is only a treatment for subfertility and not a direct treatment of RM.

The second indication for recommending IVF/ICSI to a woman with a diagnosis of RM is if she presents with a history of only biochemical pregnancies/PULs. As reviewed in Chapter 12, we believe that the majority of women with such a history have indeed had repeated spontaneously resorbed tubal pregnancies due to subtotal tubal damage and IVF/ICSI is therefore the obvious treatment option. In our clinic, more than 50% of patients with this clinical pattern will succeed to have a live birth after one to two IVF/ICSI attempts.

In conclusion, the treatments that have been reviewed in this chapter are potentially efficient treatments but they have so far not been adequately tested in RCTs in RM patients. They should therefore not be used for treating RM patients in clinical practice before these RCTs have been completed.

> ### ★ TIPS AND TRICKS
>
> Women with a history of a series of early pregnancy losses confirmed only by a home urinary pregnancy tests should be advised to attempt pregnancy once more without IVF and if repeated early plasma hCG measurements and ultrasound confirm that the pregnancy again ends as a PUL, the patient should be referred for IVF.

Bibliography

Calleja-Agius Jauniaux, E., Pizzey, A.R. and Muttukrishna, S. (2012) Investigation of systemic inflammatory response in first trimester pregnancy failure. *Human Reproduction*, **27**, 349–357.

Scarpellini, F. and Sbracia, M. (2009) Use og granulocyte colony-stimulating factor for the treatment of unexplained recurrent miscarriage: a randomized controlled trial. *Human Reproduction*, **24**, 2703–2708.

Tang T., Lord J.M., Norman R. *et al.* Insulin-sensitising drugs (metformin, rosiglitazone, pioglitazone, D-chiro-inositol) for women with polycystic ovary syndrome, oligo amenorrhoea and subfertility. *Cochrane Database of Systematic Reviews* 2012 5 (Art. No.: CD003053).

Winger, E.E. and Reed, J.L. (2008) Treatment with tumor necrosis factor inhibitors and intravenosu immunoglobulin improves live birth rates in women with recurrent spontaneous abortion. *American Journal of Reproductive Immunology*, **60**, 8–16.

9

Talking to Patients about Lifestyle, Behavior, and Miscarriage Risk

Ruth Bender Atik and Barbara E. Hepworth-Jones

The Miscarriage Association, Wakefield, UK

Introduction

Around one in five pregnancies ends in miscarriage, most commonly in the first trimester. Even so, many women experiencing their first miscarriage will be shocked and bewildered that this has happened and have little idea of how common this is.

Miscarriage is a subject not commonly discussed and women (and their partners) are likely to have read little about it in the popular pregnancy publications. Even widely read sources of information say little or nothing about miscarriage, despite its high incidence, perhaps from the mistaken belief that it might upset women unnecessarily.

Women who have previously experienced miscarriage will generally be only too aware of the possibility that it may happen again and may be anxious to take any possible action to prevent another loss. They may have researched miscarriage on the Internet and have a very misleading impression of what changes to lifestyle and behavior may be appropriate.

In every case, it is important to talk to patients in a realistic way about miscarriage. Healthcare professionals cannot and should not pretend that miscarriage is uncommon or ignore it; it is a sad but inevitable part of the cycle of life. Talking to patients about lifestyle, behavior, and miscarriage risk allows women to appreciate their own risk of miscarriage and take simple steps to reduce some of that risk.

Facts or feelings? In order to talk to patients in a realistic and helpful way, the doctor must combine three things:

- A sound knowledge of the facts of miscarriage – incidence, causes, tests, and treatments
- A commitment to keeping that knowledge updated
- An understanding of the emotional and social impact of miscarriage on patient and partner

A Sound Knowledge of the Facts

There is both a wealth and a paucity of knowledge about miscarriage: the role for the doctor is to be clear about what is fact and what is fiction, and to convey this clearly to

Recurrent Pregnancy Loss, First Edition. Edited by Ole B. Christiansen.
© 2014 John Wiley & Sons, Ltd. Published 2014 by John Wiley & Sons, Ltd.

the patient, in order to minimize unnecessary anxiety and maximize the opportunity for a future healthy pregnancy. The doctor needs to know, and to be able to cite the evidence for:

The incidence of miscarriage:
- Single/sporadic miscarriage (and its definition: note that the U.S. definition of miscarriage is pregnancy loss up to 20, rather than 24 weeks gestation)
- Recurrent miscarriage (and its definition: note that some countries define this as two or more consecutive miscarriages)
- First versus second trimester miscarriage
- Key factors affecting the incidence (e.g., maternal age)

Causes of miscarriage:
- Known causes, identifiable through investigations, and their relative importance
- Possible causes/contributing factors
- Factors that have **not been shown** to affect risk
- Factors **known** not to affect risk

Tests/investigations:
- Which investigations to carry out and when (see the Royal College of Obstetricians and Gynaecologists greentop guidelines)
- Which investigations are **not** likely to be useful

Treatments:
- Treatments for specific causes, where backed up by sound research evidence; their benefits and risks
- Treatments based on anecdotal rather than sound research evidence
- Treatments being investigated as part of an ongoing randomized controlled trial
- Treatments that may be positively harmful

A Commitment to Keeping Knowledge Updated

Medical knowledge and practice change regularly and the field of miscarriage is no exception. It is certain that patients will be acutely aware of "new information" on causes and treatments reported in the press, in addition to what they are told by family and friends. It is therefore crucial for the doctor to keep abreast of new developments, new and ongoing research, changes in guidelines and recommended practice, whether from the Royal College of Obstetricians and Gynaecologists, the Department of Health, or National Institute for Health and Care Excellence.

Understanding the Emotional and Social Impact of Miscarriage

The impact of miscarriage should not be underestimated. Whatever the scientific, legal, and/or religious perspective, many women (and their partners too) experience miscarriage as the loss of a baby, the loss of hopes, plans and expectations, of what might have been.

That is by no means always the case – others will view miscarriage as a blip in their pregnancy history, while for some it may come as a relief. But for many if not most, miscarriage at any gestation is a significant and distressing experience. Feelings of grief and loss are common, along with other somatic expressions of distress, and it may be weeks or months before they begin to recover and feel able to move forward.

This can be even more pronounced for women with recurrent miscarriage (RM) and for their partners. It can be increasingly difficult to recover emotionally from their losses and to feel positive about trying again. Many talk of losing confidence in themselves, both at home and at work. Some report symptoms of depression and relationship and sexual problems. Social and cultural/religious expectations can add pressure to either partner:

I feel a failure as a woman, a failure as a wife and a failure as a mother

Any useful discussion about miscarriage must take account of these social and emotional factors. An awareness of and sensitivity to the patient's feelings will create the best possible circumstances for clear and well-remembered communication.

The importance of information following miscarriage

Clear and accurate information is important for most women who have miscarried and for their partners. It can help them come to terms with their loss, to understand more about what has happened, and to cope with the anxieties and uncertainties of a further pregnancy. Emotional reactions to miscarriage vary widely and so will coping strategies. For some people, information that enables them to actively change factors over which there may be at least some measure of control, may provide a coping strategy. Focusing on, for example, eating a healthy diet, taking vitamins, reaching a BMI of at least 18.5 if underweight, or delaying trying to become pregnant until stressful events are over may provide a sense of control. This measure of control may be fragile; it may be necessary to provide additional information and support (or signpost appropriate sources) in the event of threatened or actual pregnancy loss or RM.

Timing

Preconceptually

The ideal time to discuss miscarriage risk is, of course, before your patient becomes pregnant again. If your patient is invited to a follow-up appointment after her miscarriage, as indeed she should, she is likely to expect answers to key questions:

- Why has this happened (again)?
- What can you do to find out the cause?
- Is it my fault? Was it something I did or should have done?
- What treatment can I have next time? (or Why did the treatment not work?)
- What can I do differently next time?

While you may wish to focus on further investigations and possible treatment, this is also the perfect opportunity to include advice and information on lifestyle and behavior, for three main reasons:

1. It could reduce the miscarriage risk for any patient, whether or not there are other underlying causes identified.
2. If the next pregnancy miscarries, with or without treatment, the patient and her partner can be reassured that that they had done all they could to reduce the risk.
3. She may conceive before she has any investigations or their results.

In Early Pregnancy

Pregnancy after RM is generally a time of high anxiety and patients are likely to search widely for any information, advice, or treatment that appears to promise, or improve the chances of success. This is the opportunity for you to talk through that information and help your patient understand the difference between evidence-based data and medical knowledge on the one hand, and myth, misunderstanding and misleading advertising and/or promises on the other.

Discussing the causes of miscarriage

The causes of sporadic and recurrent miscarriage are detailed elsewhere in this book, so we will not repeat them here. It is crucial, however, to bear in mind that patients with RM generally assume:

- that there is a single identifiable cause for their losses
- that investigations will identify this cause
- that there will be a treatment to prevent it causing a future miscarriage

They tend **not** to realize:

- that miscarriage can be multifactorial
- that consecutive miscarriages may have different causes – and crucially:
- that the most common cause, that of chance or random chromosome abnormalities, can happen in any pregnancy, despite any other treatment given

Questions may include:

Can I Be Referred for Tests?

The RCOG Green-top guidelines indicate when and which tests should be conducted in the event of RM. Many patients find it hard to accept the usual protocol of investigations after three miscarriages and seek medical investigations after one or two miscarriages.

It is generally agreed that earlier investigations are appropriate only if there are specific reasons, such as:

- indications of a clotting, autoimmune or chromosome disorder, based on patient and/or family history
- advancing maternal age (as waiting increases the miscarriage risk)
- a history of infertility or subfertility (where time taken to conceive could increase both risk and distress)
- after one or two second trimester losses.

Where there are no such extenuating circumstances, reassurance should be given that the chances of a successful pregnancy are still very high and discussion initiated about risk factors and giving the next pregnancy the best possible chance of success. This will enable women to take some measure of control over their next pregnancy.

It is important to remember that patients may take a dim view of this logic. They may feel that while one miscarriage was simply unlucky, there must be a cause if they have two or more – it cannot be pure chance. (We talk about how to explain risk and chance later.) Patients may not be able to comprehend why they should have to risk another miscarriage in order to "qualify" for investigations.

> *They did the tests after my third miscarriage and it turns out I have APS [antiphospholipid syndrome], so they'll give me aspirin and heparin next time. But if they'd tested me after my first miscarriage, I could have avoided losing two babies.*

It might be difficult to disagree with this assertion – it is certainly true that earlier testing, diagnosis, and treatment **might** have prevented this patient's second and third miscarriages, unless either was caused by something else, such a chromosomal abnormality.

The honest response lies in a combination of the statistics of chance – and the limited resources of the NHS.

Chance
Miscarriage is, of course, sadly common, affecting anything from 15% to 20% of pregnancies, depending on how it is defined. Most are caused by random (or chance) chromosome abnormalities. Statistically, the chance of two miscarriages is approximately $0.2 \times 0.2 = 0.04$ (4%) and of three miscarriages, approximately $0.04 \times 0.2 = 0.008$, or just under 1%.

In fact, the incidence of RM (three or more miscarriages) is around 2%, which suggests that approximately half of RM is caused by random chance and half has a specific cause (although currently, not every cause can be diagnosed and even if it can be, there may be no treatment available). Although the probability is not precisely the same (2.8%), you might explain RM as the equivalent of throwing three dice and getting the same number on each die – rare, but possible.

From the patient's perspective, however, this may not suffice. The APS patient mentioned earlier would discount this, in retrospect, because earlier testing may well have prevented one or both of her subsequent miscarriages. The patient who has had one or two miscarriages and is as yet untested, however, is – from a purely statistical perspective – in a different boat. Nevertheless, statistics may not make sense to her, since having investigations now could at the very least rule some problems out. The reason she is not offered tests is:

Limited resources
If investigations were to be carried out routinely after two consecutive miscarriages, the costs to the NHS would soar. If the NHS funding pot were limitless, this might be considered a good use of funds, but for the foreseeable future, it is clear that the protocols are unlikely to change. It is, perhaps, not only wise but fair to explain this to

patients. They may take the decision to seek help in the private sector, which may or may not be helpful, depending on the skills and, experience of the doctor, and the evidence base of the investigations and treatments offered.

Will the Tests Give me Clear Answers?

For those being referred for investigations, it is crucial to provide clear information about the likely outcomes in order to help reduce unrealistic expectations. Most women or couples referred for investigations will expect tests to reveal the cause of their miscarriages and to indicate an appropriate treatment to prevent recurrence. Many are disappointed if, as is common, no cause is identified. While their distress is understandable – they are looking for answers and solutions and the doctor is not providing them – they can be greatly supported by the clear explanation of two key facts:

PATIENT ADVICE

If all tests results are negative, you can help your patients by explaining that:

1. Having a specific problem identified is more likely to mean an increased, rather than a decreased risk.
2. Having **no** cause identified is actually the best news for future pregnancies.

Some patients will find this information hard to accept, and it may help to refer them to written information, which confirms this (RCOG patient information, Miscarriage Association leaflets). Again, discussing risk factors and, in particular, focusing on areas where changes may realistically be made is a practical course of action in this situation.

They didn't find anything wrong. But if there's nothing wrong with me, why do I keep losing babies?

When Can I Try Again?

There is evidence that the interval between pregnancies does not affect outcome, and indeed, a short interval may even improve outcome, so there is no need to advise that women wait for a specified time after a miscarriage before trying to become pregnant again. The best advice is that your patient should try when she feels ready, physically and emotionally, with the caveats below.

⚜ CAUTION

There are three exceptions to the general guide on when to try again:

- Women diagnosed with a molar pregnancy, who will be under the care of a specialist center and will receive individual advice about when they may safely become pregnant again

- Women treated with methotrexate following ectopic pregnancy, who will be advised to wait (usually) 3 months before trying again
- Women undergoing specific investigations for RM, who should wait until these are completed in case they indicate action before or during the next pregnancy

When Should I Have a Scan?

Seeing a heartbeat on a scan is very reassuring, as it indicates a high probability of a successful pregnancy. However, not seeing a heartbeat in early pregnancy does not necessarily indicate miscarriage. Women may for example have ovulated late in their cycle, or may have a longer cycle than usual, so the pregnancy may not be as advanced as dates suggest.

If a heartbeat does not show on a very early scan, this may indicate that the pregnancy is not viable, but it may simply be too early to see, and a repeat scan will then be needed to confirm the diagnosis. This will raise anxiety, especially for women who have had previous miscarriage diagnosed by a scan, which failed to show a heartbeat.

Assuming a reasonably regular cycle of about 28 days, it may be preferable to arrange for the first scan around 7 weeks after LMP, when a heartbeat should be seen in a viable pregnancy. Even then, if a heartbeat cannot be seen, a repeat scan a week later should be performed to confirm that the pregnancy has miscarried. Whilst repeat scans are good practice to ensure that potentially viable pregnancies are not treated as miscarriages, this is a time of high anxiety for women and they may require information and support.

Women with a history of ectopic pregnancy will require an early scan to confirm the location of the pregnancy and it is important to explain that not seeing a heartbeat at, say, 5–6 weeks gestation, is to be expected and perfectly normal.

Does the Treatment I Chose for My Previous Miscarriage Affect My Future Risk?

Women may ask if the method of treatment of a previous miscarriage affects their risk of miscarriage in future pregnancies. There is evidence that the choice of surgical, medical, or expectant management of a previous miscarriage does not affect future pregnancy outcome.

I am Feeling Stressed – Is This a Problem?

There is increasing evidence that emotional well-being may be related to risk of miscarriage. Stress and traumatic events appear to increase risk, while feeling relaxed and happy appears to decrease the risk. Risk appears greater with an increasing number of stressful or traumatic events, such separation or divorce, serious financial problems, serious illness, or death of someone close.

It may be appropriate to suggest waiting before conception in order to reduce the risk of miscarriage as much as possible, for example after a specific event such as a bereavement; or it may be possible to suggest changes to reduce stress, for example changing to a less stressful job. When advising in early pregnancy or where the stress is unavoidable or likely to persist for a long period, it is important to put the risk in to

> **QUICK QUIZ 1**
>
> After three miscarriages, Mr. and Mrs. Brown's investigations all showed normal results. The consultant has told them that this is very good news but Mrs. Brown does not see it that way at all and seems very upset.
>
> - Why does the consultant see these results as good news?
> - Why might Mrs. Brown see it differently?
> - What expectations might she have had?
> - Is there anything you can say that might change her view?
>
> *Note*: suggested answers are at the end of this chapter.

context and to highlight other ways to minimize risk, for example, taking vitamins and eating a healthy diet. It must be remembered that pregnancy after miscarriage will itself be stressful and particularly so after RM.

Discussing the concept of risk

The concept of risk is generally poorly understood, yet it is essential in order for relevant information to be imparted and acted upon. It is also crucial in reducing guilt and self-blame, should the pregnancy miscarry.

It is important to stress that increased risk does not equate to cause. It may be helpful to give relevant examples of increased risk and cause, for example, heavy smokers who never develop smoking-related diseases and light smokers who do. This is further complicated in the case of miscarriage as it is usually not possible to find a definite cause, so it is generally not possible to correlate miscarriage with a specific risk factor.

Setting realistic expectations

> **★ TIPS AND TRICKS**
>
> - Be realistic. It is possible to take action on some risk factors such as diet, but many risk factors cannot be changed, such as age and history of previous miscarriage
> - Many causes of miscarriage, such as random chromosomal abnormalities, cannot be controlled

One of the most important factors is previous reproductive history, a key indicator of risk (Table 9.1). Even after three miscarriages, a patient is more likely to have a successful pregnancy than to miscarry. However, it is important to remember that probabilities are scant consolation to a woman who has miscarried – for her, this pregnancy is a 100% failure.

Many of the potential and actual risk factors for miscarriage cannot be changed, so it is important to balance discussion of these factors with discussion about factors over which there may be control. This will help to provide a realistic picture of the likelihood of success of subsequent pregnancies.

Advice for the best possible chance of a healthy pregnancy

Recent good-quality research has highlighted several biological, behavioral, and life-style risk factors for first trimester miscarriage (see Maconochie *et al.* 2007). Discussion should be tailored to the individual patient and includes sensitive but realistic discussion of immutable factors such as parental age and pregnancy history, summarized in Tables 9.1 and 9.2. It may be valuable to concentrate discussion on factors over which there may be control, summarized in Table 9.3. Women may also find it reassuring to discuss factors that commonly cause concern, but for which there is no evidence of effect on risk, summarized in Table 9.4.

Table 9.1 Previous Reproductive History and Risk of Pregnancy Loss

Reproductive Status	Percentage Risk of Pregnancy Loss
No previous pregnancy loss	15–20% (depending on how pregnancy is defined)
Miscarriage	
One miscarriage	20%
Two miscarriages	28%
Three miscarriages	43%
Ectopic Pregnancy	
One ectopic pregnancy	2–10%
Two ectopic pregnancies	16–20%
Molar Pregnancy	
One molar pregnancy	under 2%
Two molar pregnancies	17%

Table 9.2 Factors Affecting the Risk of Miscarriage and Over Which There is Little or No Control

Factors Associated with Increased Risk
Being over 35. The risk is greatest for women over 40, who are five times more likely to miscarry than those aged 25–29
Having one or more previous miscarriages (see Table 9.1)
Having a termination for nonmedical reasons
Time to conceive. Women who take more than a year to conceive are twice as likely to miscarry as those who conceive within 3 months
Fertility problems, particularly those affecting the fallopian tubes
Assisted conception
Father over 45
Factors Associated with Reduced Risk
A previous live birth
A planned pregnancy
Nausea in early pregnancy

Table 9.3 Factors Affecting the Risk of Miscarriage and Over Which there *may* be Control

Science Revisited
Factors Associated with Increased Risk
Being underweight, with a body mass index of less than 18.5 before pregnancy
Regular/heavy drinking. Risks are highest for women who drink every day and/or more than 14 units a week
Stress. Women under continuing stress (e.g., having a very stressful or demanding job) are more likely to miscarry. It may be possible to reduce some sources of stress, for example, moving jobs.
Caffeine
Being overweight or obese
Factors Associated with Reduced Risk
Taking vitamins, particularly containing folic acid, iron or multivitamins
Eating fruit and vegetables, dairy products, and chocolate on most days, and (possibly) eating fish or white meat twice weekly or more
Feeling happy, relaxed, and in control
Factors Where Evidence is Contradictory or Weak and Where Precaution may be Advised
Smoking
Strenuous exercise

Table 9.4 Factors that Do Not Appear to Affect the Risk of Miscarriage

Science Revisited
Factors Which do not Appear to Affect the Risk of Miscarriage
Pregnancy order, that is, whether it is a first or later pregnancy
Having a short interval since the last pregnancy
Having pre-eclampsia in a previous pregnancy
Eating red meat, eggs, soya products, and sugar substitutes
Working full time
Work involving moderate physical activity
Partner's alcohol consumption in the 3 months before conception
Partner's smoking either before conception or during the pregnancy
Sex – as long as there is no bleeding
Air travel

There are a very few occupational hazards that are harmful in early pregnancy and may increase the risk of miscarriage. Other than those who work with toxic chemicals and heavy metals, women may be reassured; those who do work in a risky environment should have been made well aware of any potential risk by their employers, who have a duty of care to their employees.

For women in occupations where there is exposure to chemicals, many employers will offer to move women planning a pregnancy to another area of work to avoid exposure, even in the absence of firm evidence that such exposure is harmful. If they are in doubt, refer women to their Occupational Health or Human Resources department /officer or Union for more specific information.

Studies on risk factors for miscarriage generally involve women who have had one or two first trimester miscarriages, as they form the majority of those miscarrying. There is no evidence that advice based on these studies does not apply equally to those experiencing RM or second trimester loss and there is no specific additional information on risk factors in these situations.

PATIENT ADVICE

The following checklist summarizes general advice that may be given to patients to reduce the risk of miscarriage:

- Maintain a healthy bodyweight (BMI between 18.5 and 30 and preferably 25).
- Avoid regular/heavy drinking, especially drinking every day. The best advice is to avoid alcohol completely to reduce risks to your pregnancy and to your baby's health after birth.
- Avoid unnecessary stress and focus on what will make you feel happy, relaxed and in control, such as making time for activities you enjoy, having a chocolate treat, walking or other gentle exercise, and talking to supportive friends.
- Avoid or reduce caffeine intake, particularly the high levels found in coffee, cola, and energy drinks.
- Take vitamins designed for prepregnancy/early pregnancy, containing folic acid, iron and multivitamins.
- Eat a healthy diet, with fruit and vegetables and dairy products most days and fish or white meat at least twice a week.
- Avoid smoking and illicit drug use.
- Avoid strenuous exercise.

Risk and cause

PEARLS TO TAKE HOME

Help your patient understand that risk is not the same as cause

For those who have previously experienced miscarriage, the corollary of giving advice about the next pregnancy is that women may then wonder if *not* following that advice caused or contributed to their miscarriage(s). Be prepared to go over the concept of risk again and stress that risk is not the same as cause. Discuss the fact that each individual factor has only a small influence; it is the collective effect that is important and women should not worry unduly if one or two factors cannot be or were not changed.

> **QUICK QUIZ 2**
>
> Ms Green is 28 and has had three miscarriages. All investigations show normal results, but she is worried that one or more of the following might have caused the miscarriages. How would you advise her?
>
> - She had a termination before these pregnancies: it was the wrong time for a baby.
> - She drinks a lot of coffee – it helps her cope with a busy work schedule.
> - Her work means she has to travel a lot, usually by air.
>
> *Note*: suggested answers are at the end of this chapter

Talking to patients you have advised, after another miscarriage

I did everything I should have – healthy diet, no alcohol or smoking, taking folic acid etc. I know there's no order of how things happen in life, but after doing everything right, it just feels so unfair.

The advice that you give to women and their partners will give the best possible chance of a healthy pregnancy, but it cannot guarantee success. Even after taking steps to reduce risk, there is always still a significant chance of another miscarriage, hence the importance of setting realistic expectations. Should another miscarriage happen, you can provide reassurance that your patients took action to reduce risk, perhaps even reducing every risk over which they had control.

As always with miscarriage, there will be a wide range of reactions and feelings in this situation. Some women may actually be relieved that they have had a third miscarriage and now "qualify" for investigations. Others may be apprehensive or even fearful, when they have done everything possible to reduce risk and yet it still happened again. The unspoken thought might be "I may never have a baby." It is important to refer women to appropriate sources of information and support.

This may be the time to review the lifestyle advice you previously gave, to see if anything has changed. For example, you may have previously discounted advising about reducing stress by considering a change in job, as this may be very difficult to achieve. However, in view of another miscarriage, the time may now be right to discuss this possibility.

Prospects may seem bleak after another miscarriage, but you may reassure your patients that there is still a good chance that the next pregnancy will be successful; further information may be found in Table 9.1. And following the lifestyle advice is equally important for the next pregnancy, to give the best possible chance of success.

The importance of good care

> **PEARLS TO TAKE HOME**
>
> There is good evidence that "tender loving care" for couples with idiopathic RM can improve pregnancy outcomes.

In two studies looking at the provision of "tender loving care" for couples with idiopathic RM, the offer of open access for scanning and support in pregnancy after miscarriage was often enough in itself; it was not necessarily taken up. Support could include preconception care and advice and someone to talk to: health professional, counselor, or support organization.

Good care also requires the use of appropriate medical terminology, along with explanations for those not familiar with it. It is important to bear in mind that some clinical terms can cause great distress and even anger. It is not acceptable to use the term "abortion" for miscarriage, despite its historical clinical prevalence. To the lay person, "abortion" means the elective termination of pregnancy and while they may have no theoretical objections to that procedure, they are likely to be distressed and even angered at its use in their situation. "Miscarriage" (qualified by adjectives such as recurrent, delayed, early, late, etc.) is easily understood and well accepted.

Similarly, the terms "products of conception," "blighted ovum," and "cervical incompetence" can also cause distress. While all of us are, by definition, products of conception, most women consider their pregnancy as a baby rather than a product, and this is especially likely for miscarriage patients. In a recent poll of 1280 patients and professionals, 76% indicated that the term ERPC (evacuation of retained products of conception) needed changing, and the overwhelming preference (80%) was for "surgical management of miscarriage."

The terms "blighted ovum" and "cervical incompetence" both imply blame. Alternatives to the first are "early embryo loss" or "delayed miscarriage" (the term, "empty sac" may also be used but requires clear explanation – the obvious question it evokes is "so where has it gone?"). Cervical incompetence is better described as cervical weakness.

It is helpful to take your cue from parents when it comes to describing the embryo or fetus (if there was one). Although a small number will refer to an embryo or fetus or just to "the pregnancy", most will use the term "baby." You should aim to do likewise, even if you believe this to be inaccurate (e.g., in a molar pregnancy or early embryo loss).

Even though it will require careful explanation, the term "molar pregnancy" is likely to be more acceptable to patients than "gestational trophoblastic disease." The term "ectopic pregnancy" is generally accepted, though at different stages it may be referred to as a PUL or a tubal pregnancy.

In general, the term "pregnancy loss" can be used to cover miscarriage, ectopic and molar pregnancy.

⚓ CAUTION

The following terms, whilst medically accurate, commonly cause distress and should be avoided:

Abortion – spontaneous, recurrent, or missed
Recurrent or habitual aborter
Products of conception/retained products of conception
Blighted ovum
Cervical incompetence

Sources of information and support

Whilst healthcare professionals are the most important source of information and support about pregnancy loss, the time available to spend with each individual patient is limited and it is important to be able to refer women and their partners to additional reliable sources of information and support, if they wish. Time spent with the patient may then focus on specific and tailored lifestyle advice, as already discussed.

The Miscarriage Association, for example, offers support through a telephone helpline, e-mail, local peer support, a website including online leaflets, moderated online discussion forums and Facebook pages. There are many other sources of Internet support such as unmoderated chat rooms and discussion forums. Some hospitals may organize support groups for pregnancy loss or offer counseling services. There are also a number of books on pregnancy loss.

Information on and support for pregnancy loss may readily be found on the Internet, but caution should be exercised as some information is misleading and unmoderated discussion forums may also give incorrect or even biased advice. However, there are reliable sources of information. The following is an excerpt from the Miscarriage Association leaflet "Thinking about another pregnancy":

"CAN I REDUCE MY RISK OF ANOTHER MISCARRIAGE?"

There may be things you can do and we will explain about some of these in the next sections. But it is important to know that however hard you try, you cannot completely rule out the chance of another miscarriage.

It is helpful to know the difference between a risk and a cause. Take alcohol for example: we know that regular or heavy drinking in pregnancy raises the **risk** of miscarriage; but even if you drank a lot in your last pregnancy, that does not mean it **caused** your miscarriage. Even so, you might decide to cut down or stop drinking altogether next time.

So what can I do?

You and your partner may be able to take steps to improve your general health, diet, and lifestyle. This can make a difference to your chances of getting pregnant and having a healthy pregnancy.

We do not know why these improvements make a difference, or why they help some people more than others. As we said earlier, there are no guarantees. But you might find the information in the next pages helpful.

It was quite a comfort when the midwife said that lots of women who have two miscarriages go on to have a good next pregnancy, but that doesn't change the fact that that might not be me! Statistics are all very well but the chances for you personally are either 100% or 0%.

Additional sources of information and support that might be useful for you and your patients are listed at the end of this chapter.

> ★ **TIPS AND TRICKS**
>
> - Tender loving care, such as the offer of an early scan, improves the chance of a successful pregnancy
> - Listen to your patient and her partner and know where to source additional information and further support

When the trying stops

There can come a point at which patients with a history of repeated miscarriage make the decision to stop trying for another pregnancy. They may look at adoption or fostering, or to focus on any existing child or children; or they may accept that they will remain childless and move toward a different future from the one they had planned and hoped for.

Deciding not to try again is a life-changing choice and couples may make and "unmake" this decision many times, perhaps over many months or even years. Crucially, it is a decision for each woman or couple alone. You may want to support them in thinking about the possibility of stopping, but you should not assume that you know what is best.

> ✋ **CAUTION**
>
> <u>Do not</u> advise your patients to stop trying to have a baby, unless there are strong medical reasons to avoid another pregnancy.
>
> <u>Do</u> acknowledge how distressing repeated miscarriage can be, and consider asking if they have ever thought of stopping trying.
>
> <u>Do</u> read and perhaps recommend the Miscarriage Association leaflet **When the Trying Stops**, freely available on our website.

Summary

Talking to pre-pregnancy or pre-gnant patients about lifestyle, behavior, and miscarriage risk is appropriate, whether or not there is a history of miscarriage. For those who have had RM, this is even more crucial. Providing realistic advice regarding risk can not only enable women and their partners to take practical steps to reduce that risk, but also offer reassurance. In addition, it can ensure that women and their partners have realistic expectations about their chances of a successful pregnancy.

> **ANSWERS TO QUICK QUIZ 1**
>
> After three miscarriages, Mr. and Mrs. Brown's investigations all showed normal results. The consultant has told them that this is very good news but Mrs. Brown does not see it that way at all and seems very upset.

Reasons that she might be upset with these results.

- She wants to know why she miscarried – and she still does not have any answers.
- If there is no medical problem diagnosed and therefore no treatment, then she is just as likely as before to miscarry again.
- If there is no medical explanation, it must be her fault that she is miscarrying.

What to say that might help to change her view.

- That you understand how difficult it is not to know why she has been miscarrying.
- That you appreciate how hard it is to consider another pregnancy without any treatment that might improve the outcome.
- That none of the things the tests might have found would have been good news.
- That there is evidence that she has a good chance of having a healthy pregnancy without any further intervention.

ANSWERS TO QUICK QUIZ 2

Ms Green is 28 and has had three miscarriages. All investigations show normal results, but she is worried that one or more of the following might have caused the miscarriages. How would you advise her?

Previous TOP for nonmedical reasons and consuming caffeine are both associated with a higher risk of miscarriage. Stress at work is also associated with increased miscarriage risk. But:

- Despite the increased risk, that does not mean these factors caused the miscarriages.
- She cannot do anything to change the termination history, but she could drink less coffee in a future pregnancy.
- She does not say she is stressed at work and flying is not associated with an increased risk. Ask – and if work is stressful, perhaps discuss possible strategies to reduce this in the next pregnancy.

Further sources of information and support

The Miscarriage Association	www.miscarriageassociation.org.uk Information and support on miscarriage, ectopic and molar pregnancy
Ectopic Pregnancy Trust	www.ectopic.org.uk
SANDS	www.uk-sands.org The stillbirth and neonatal death charity

Bibiliography

Liddle, H.S., Pattinson, N.S. and Zanderigo, A. (1991) *Recurrent miscarriage – outcome after supportive care in early pregnancy. Australian Journal of Obstetrics & Gynaecology*, **31** (4), 320–322.

Maconochie, N., Doyle, P., Prior, S. and Simmons, R. (2007) *Risk factors for first trimester miscarriage: results from a UK-population-based case-control study. BJOG*, **114** (2), 170–186.

Royal College of Obstetricians and Gynaecologists. *The investigation and treatment of couples with recurrent first-trimester and second-trimester miscarriage.* (Green-top Guidelines No. 17). Royal College of Obstetricians and Gynaecologists, 2011.

10

Endocrine and Ultrasonic Surveillance of Pregnancies in Patients with Recurrent Miscarriage

Adjoa Appiah and Jemma Johns

Early Pregnancy and Gynaecology Assessment Unit, King's College Hospital, London, UK

Introduction

There is a great deal of published literature on the management of couples with recurrent pregnancy loss (RPL), both preconception and during the first trimester; however, improvements in live birth rates have not been forthcoming in randomized controlled trials (RCT) of potential treatments for couples with idiopathic RPL. The only treatment recognized to improve the live birth rate is the use of aspirin and heparin in the treatment of women with antiphospholipid syndrome. This chapter examines the role of assessment and monitoring of pregnancies at increased risk of miscarriage in the first trimester. In particular, it examines the evidence surrounding endocrine and ultrasound surveillance of these pregnancies.

The risk of first trimester miscarriage increases with each pregnancy loss, approaching 35% in parous and 45% in nulliparous women after three or more miscarriages. Confirmation of a new pregnancy can be an emotionally challenging time for couples who have experienced RPL. In the early stages of a new pregnancy, many couples may opt to keep the news to themselves until the pregnancy is more advanced for fear of another miscarriage, protecting themselves, family, and friends from further emotional trauma. Couples will also sometimes avoid healthcare professionals for fear of wasting their time and in order not to build up their hopes, only to experience yet another miscarriage. The majority however will present early to early pregnancy units (EPU), seeking reassurance that the pregnancy is ongoing. At this initial assessment, anxiety levels are high and healthcare professionals need to be experienced at assessing early pregnancies accurately and with sensitivity at this difficult time.

Early pregnancy-related fear has been associated with later complications during pregnancy and delivery. For couples with RPL, preconception counseling in the RPL clinic should include encouragement to seek early support when they become pregnant again. Couples with idiopathic RPL have a good chance of a live birth in

Recurrent Pregnancy Loss, First Edition. Edited by Ole B. Christiansen.
© 2014 John Wiley & Sons, Ltd. Published 2014 by John Wiley & Sons, Ltd.

subsequent pregnancies with supportive care alone from 6 weeks of pregnancy, with the live birth rate being estimated to be as high as 75%.

This chapter aims to review the evidence for the use of endocrine and sonographic investigations in the assessment of early pregnancy, including its role in establishing the location of early pregnancy and predicting pregnancy outcome with particular reference to RPL. We will also attempt to assess the evidence for the role of "supportive care" for couples who have experienced RPL, in subsequent pregnancies. The treatment of specific disorders is discussed in detail elsewhere in this publication and will not be discussed here; however their management in the first trimester is often similar.

The role of endocrine surveillance

The pregnancy hormones play a very important role in adapting a woman's body to childbirth and lactation and maintaining a suitable environment for fetal growth (Figure 10.1). Inevitably, this has led to extensive research, looking for fetoplacental markers to predict both early and late pregnancy outcomes.

Of the hormones specific to pregnancy, human chorionic gonadotropin (hCG) and progesterone have been those most studied and remain the most promising in early pregnancy, both to assess their role in predicting the likelihood of miscarriage and in the management of miscarriage and pregnancy of unknown location (PUL).

The majority of pregnant women with RPL have no pre-existing endocrine abnormalities; however historically endocrine factors have been implicated in the etiology of RPL. Of these, thyroid abnormalities and diabetes have been the most thoroughly investigated. More recently, a clearer understanding of the endocrine abnormalities in polycystic ovarian syndrome (PCOS) has resulted in interest in treatment of insulin resistance in women with subfertility and miscarriage related to this disorder.

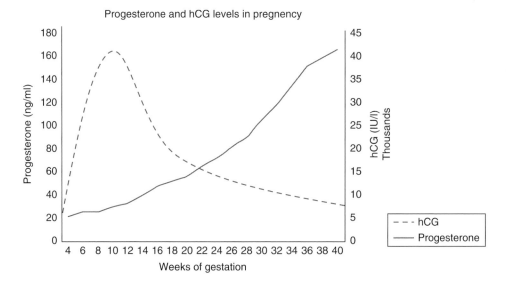

Figure 10.1 Serum progesterone and βhCG levels in a normal singleton pregnancy. (Conversion of progesterone from ng/ml to nmol/l is a factor of 3.18).

Prediction of miscarriage

The role of serum markers for the prediction of outcome in early pregnancy in women with or without a history of RPL has been extensively investigated, with serum βhCG and serum progesterone being the best recognized. The vast majority of data is from women with sporadic pregnancy loss and may not always be applicable to the RPL population. This data is also often from symptomatic pregnancies rather than women presenting for reassurance in the absence of bleeding or pain. In addition to serum βhCG and serum progesterone other serum markers such as inhibin, activin, and estradiol have been evaluated for their role in predicting the viability of an early pregnancy.

Progesterone

Progesterone is responsible for preparing the endometrium for implantation, modulating immune responses to pregnancy, and preventing the onset of uterine contractions, and it is essential for the maintenance of early pregnancy. Withdrawal of progesterone before 7 weeks gestation by removal of the corpus luteum or by using antiprogestogenic drugs has been associated with an increased risk of pregnancy loss.

The concept that failure of the corpus luteum to adequately support a pregnancy with progesterone leads to early pregnancy loss is an attractive one. Alternatively, if there is sufficient progesterone production but a poor endometrial response, this could potentially jeopardize implantation. Both these factors have been considered to play a role in the pathophysiology of luteal phase deficiency (LPD). This has led to the use of progesterone supplementation in early pregnancy, both in threatened miscarriage and RPL. Difficulties in classification and diagnosis of LPD have, however, led to much controversy over the existence of this disorder.

The role of measuring serum progesterone in the prediction of pregnancy outcome, both in asymptomatic women and those presenting with threatened miscarriage, has been extensively investigated, and its use is now established in many dedicated EPUs. Serum progesterone levels are generally lower in pregnancies destined to miscarry.

SCIENCE REVISITED

Progesterone is produced by the corpus luteum in the first 10 weeks of pregnancy and thereafter by the placenta. In normal pregnancies, levels rise after fertilization and continue increasing steadily until term.

βhCG is a glycoprotein produced by the syncytiotrophoblast and is composed of α and β subunits. Commonly used assays are for the β subunit, as the α subunit is similar in structure to follicle-stimulating hormone, luteinizing hormone, and thyrotropin. It is detected in maternal serum as early as 8 days after ovulation in a serum sample and from about 12–14 days in urine. Levels approximately double every 2 days and peak at about 10 weeks. Thereafter, there is a decline until around 20 weeks when plasma levels remain low and constant until term.

There are many assays for progesterone and βhCG, and as a result units of measure vary between laboratories.

The lowest recorded initial serum progesterone level in the presence of an intrauterine gestation sac (GS) on ultrasound, where the pregnancy was subsequently found to be ongoing, has been shown to be 12 ng/ml (38.4 nmol/l). Using a cutoff of >15 ng/ml (48 nmol/l) it is possible to predict an ongoing pregnancy with a sensitivity of 87% and specificity of 83%. More recently, a larger prospective observational study of 200 women with a mean sac diameter (MSD, where the sac is measured in three orthogonal planes and averaged) of <20 mm and no embryo on transvaginal ultrasound scan (TVS) showed that the serum progesterone level was the single most powerful predictor of pregnancy outcome. At a cutoff of 25 nmol/l it was possible to predict an ongoing pregnancy with a sensitivity of 100% and specificity of 40%. In this study, there were no ongoing pregnancies where initial levels were <25 nmol/l. When serum progesterone was used in a logistic regression model using multiple variables (MSD, maternal age, and serum progesterone), the diagnosis of a viable pregnancy could be made with a sensitivity of 99.2% and specificity of 70.7%. When this model was tested in routine practice, the logistic regression model performed better than each of the individual parameters and was able to predict viability of pregnancy with reasonable accuracy.

Serum progesterone levels have been shown to have a good predictive value in women with PUL. An initial level of ≤20 nmol/l has a predictive value of about 95% for pregnancy failure. Levels greater than 25 nmol/l are likely to indicate viable pregnancy, whether intrauterine or ectopic, whereas those above 60 nmol/l are strongly associated with viability, irrespective of location. Serial serum progesterone levels have not been shown to increase the discriminatory power over and above a single measurement.

Human Chorionic Gonadotropin

The other most extensively researched pregnancy hormone is the human chorionic gonadotropin (hCG). Several studies have reported the association between low initial serum βhCG and pregnancy failure in women with and without vaginal bleeding in the first trimester.

The use of serial serum βhCG levels is routine in managing women who have a positive pregnancy test but have no evidence of an intra- or extrauterine pregnancy on transvaginal scan. Such pregnancies are known as PULs. An increase of more than 66% over 48 h is a good predictor of a viable pregnancy. However, the slowest rate of rise associated with a subsequent viable intrauterine pregnancy has been reported as 53% in 48 h. This data will have to be interpreted with caution in asymptomatic women. Despite this, the clinical value of serum βhCG for the prediction of outcome remains to be established and serum βhCG is not able to accurately determine pregnancy location. Its role is principally in the monitoring of PULs and ectopic pregnancies that have been managed by salpingotomy, expectant and medical methods.

> ### ✋ CAUTION
>
> It is essential that serum levels of βhCG and progesterone are interpreted in the context of ultrasound findings and clinical history. Discriminatory zones for serum βhCG are of limited value and should not be used in isolation. Serum βhCG tells us how much trophoblastic tissue is present and serum progesterone indicates the viability of such tissue. Neither will identify the location of the pregnancy and in addition assessment of symptomatic early pregnancies should be made in the context of the clinical history and ultrasound findings.

The role of ultrasound surveillance

With the advent of transvaginal ultrasound in the 1970s the diagnosis of pregnancy can be made approximately 1–2 weeks earlier than with the transabdominal probe. Women with RPL are encouraged to attend for an early scan and the optimum time for this is generally accepted to be around 6 weeks gestation.

The ability to assess pregnancies early has inevitably led to an increase in the incidence of PUL, and it is essential that ultrasound assessment is made in the context of a clinical history which takes into account an accurate menstrual and reproductive history. Performing the scan too early will not only result in extensive investigation of a PUL but will inevitably result in increased anxiety levels in this population. Knowledge of the ultrasonic landmarks in early pregnancy is essential in order to avoid unnecessary delay in diagnosis or misdiagnosis of a miscarriage or ectopic pregnancy.

EVIDENCE AT A GLANCE

A prospective study of 1442 symptomatic and asymptomatic women attending for TVS scan prior to 84 days of gestation in a UK based EPU concluded that the ability to confirm viability or nonviability was related to gestational age. Prior to 35 days of gestation the commonest finding was PUL, between 35 and 41 days was an early intrauterine pregnancy of uncertain viability, and from 42 days a viable intrauterine pregnancy. Miscarriage could only be diagnosed on initial TVS after 35 days. Therefore, to reduce the number of inconclusive scans without risking morbidity from missed ectopic pregnancies, TVS should be delayed until 49 days in asymptomatic women with no previous history of ectopic pregnancy.

The gestation sac (GS) is the earliest structure identified and can be seen by 4–5 weeks gestation, where the MSD ranges from 2 to 5 mm. By 5–6 weeks the thickened decidua can be seen around the gestational sac and this is known as the double-decidua sign. The presence of the yolk sac in the fifth week confirms the diagnosis of an intrauterine pregnancy. The fetal pole is seen at about 5–6 weeks as a linear hyperechoic structure adjacent to the yolk sac (Figure 10.2). Between 5 and 7 weeks the GS and embryo grow approximately 1 mm/day. A fetal heartbeat (FH) can typically be seen with a crown rump length (CRL) of about 2 mm, but is almost always present when the embryo is 5 mm. This is the first confirmation of a viable intrauterine pregnancy. In normal pregnancy, FH increases from a mean of 110 beats per minute (bpm) at 6 weeks to a maximum of about 175 bpm at 9 weeks and decreases thereafter. In cases of known intrauterine pregnancy, viability will be uncertain in approximately 10% of women at their first visit to an EPU.

★ TIPS AND TRICKS

Due to the emotive nature of the diagnosis of miscarriage, when this is suspected on ultrasound scan a second, and preferably more senior, opinion should be sought to confirm the diagnosis. Alternatively, a rescan could be offered with a recommended minimum interval of 7 days between scans to confirm the diagnosis. The latter allows for confirmation of absent development of the pregnancy.

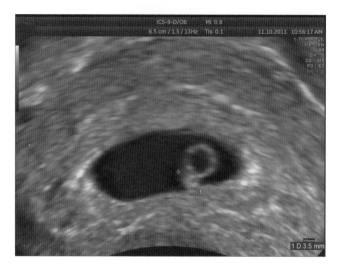

Figure 10.2 Transvaginal ultrasound picture of 6 weeks gestation. Yolk sac is seen to the right of the fetal pole (marked). A fetal heartbeat was seen during this scan.

Prediction of miscarriage

Evidence of a GS, yolk sac, and fetal pole with or without cardiac activity on the first visit and on subsequent visits have all been investigated either individually or together for their role in predicting miscarriage. A retrospective review has demonstrated that in the prediction of miscarriage there was significant contribution from a combination of CRL, FH, MSD, and yolk sac diameter, in addition to maternal factors such as age.

Once a gestational sac has been documented on ultrasound, subsequent loss of viability in the embryonic period remains around 11% in the general population. A smaller than expected CRL as a possible marker of early pregnancy failure has been well documented. In women with no history of bleeding or RPL, if an embryo has developed up to 5 mm in length on TVS, subsequent loss of viability occurs in 7.2% of cases. Loss rates drop to 3.3% for embryos of 6–10 mm and to 0.5% for embryos over 10 mm.

There is a wide range for GS size in "normal" pregnancy, and recent evidence has suggested that a single MSD or CRL measurement is not reliable enough to enable an accurate diagnosis of nonviability; in addition, there is no cutoff for MSD growth below which a viable pregnancy can be excluded. This would suggest that the current universally applied criteria for the diagnosis of miscarriage based on a single measurement of the MSD or CRL are potentially unsafe and should be abandoned. It is important to note that even normal, viable pregnancies may not measurably grow in size within 7–10 days.

On the basis of this evidence the Royal College of Obstetricians and Gynaecologists (RCOG) has recently amended its guideline on the management of early pregnancy loss in line with this finding and recommends that the diagnosis of miscarriage should be considered with an MSD ≥25 mm and no obvious yolk sac, or with a fetal pole with CRL ≥7 mm and no evidence of an FH. It is also recommended that all women are rescanned at a 7–10 days interval if there is uncertainty. The authors would suggest that the latter should probably be applied in all cases, unless there is clear evidence of previous viability.

In general, studies looking at the predictive value of FH activity on miscarriage in the general population can be divided into those examining the presence of fetal heart activity and those examining fetal heart rate in relation to outcome. A single observation of an abnormally slow heart rate does not necessarily indicate subsequent embryonic death, but a continuous decline observed within a few days interval is inevitably associated with miscarriage.

In practice, the identification of a slow fetal heart rate is not necessarily an indication to bring a woman back for a repeat scan as the prognosis is uncertain. It is difficult under these circumstances to decide when the most appropriate time would be for a repeat scan and should be determined by symptomatology in addition to previous history in the first instance. It would be reasonable to arrange a repeat scan in 7–10 days unless bleeding or worsening of presenting symptoms occurs in the interim. Deciding upon whether to inform the patient that the FHR is slower than expected should be individualized, depending upon the circumstances and clinical presentation.

Subchorionic hematoma

The finding of fluid or hematomata surrounding the gestational sac is relatively common in women with or without vaginal bleeding. The reported incidence ranges from 4% to 22%. Subchorionic hematomas appear as hypoechoic or mixed echogenic, crescent shaped structures, located between the uterine wall and the chorionic membrane. Occasionally, they can also be seen bulging into the GS and are known as "chorionic bumps." Prognosis appears to be independent of the site or size of the hematoma and is related to the occurrence of vaginal bleeding with an associated small increased risk of miscarriage.

Large hematomas seen in the first trimester and first and second trimester vaginal bleeding have been associated with premature prelabor rupture of membranes (PPROM), preterm labor or abruptio placenta in later pregnancy.

One small observational study reported a specific increase in the occurrence of intrauterine hematoma in subsequent pregnancies of women with RPL. It reported an incidence of 12% and it was noted that in this group many of the women were on anticoagulation for thrombophilia, when compared to the control group. It was also concluded that there was no statistically significant difference in adverse obstetric outcome between the group with hematomas and controls.

Vanishing twin syndrome

The idea that more twins were conceived than born has been around since the 1940s. In a multifetal pregnancy, the apparent disappearance of a previously seen GS on ultrasound scan is known as the vanishing twin syndrome (VTS), and normally results in a singleton pregnancy. The incidence is reported to be as high as 30% of all twin pregnancies following assisted conception, and is even more uncertain for spontaneous conceptions where early pregnancy scans are not done routinely prior to the nuchal scan. It can also occur in higher order multifetal pregnancies. There is no known increased risk of VTS in women with RPL.

VTS typically occurs in the first trimester and this may be because generally the risk of miscarriage is highest at this point. As with all miscarriages fetal and/or placental abnormalities have been implicated in this phenomenon, in particular those arising from chromosomal abnormalities. Increased incidence of VTS is seen with advanced maternal age, further supporting the idea of genetic abnormalities. The occurrence of VTS is not influenced by the zygosity of the twins.

The patient may be asymptomatic if it occurs in the first trimester, but others may present with pain and bleeding in early pregnancy. Generally, the surviving twin is unaffected if VTS occurs in the first trimester.

The ultrasonic appearance of VTS is variable, depending on the gestation at which the nonviable pregnancy fails. Generally, it is suspected in the presence of a second smaller empty sac adjacent to an ongoing early pregnancy. The appearance of VTS should not be confused with the presence of a subchorionic hematoma or fluid; however, differentiating them can be difficult.

First trimester screening

First trimester screening is used to determine the risk of chromosomal abnormalities such as Down's syndrome (or trisomy 21) and some fetal abnormalities such as congenital heart disease. It is well established that the risk of embryonic chromosomal abnormalities and congenital malformations in the fetuses of women with a history of RPL is generally lower than in women with sporadic miscarriages/common population. Most screening programs combine maternal age with maternal blood biochemistry and ultrasound findings in order to predict risk. The ultrasound marker used in the combined test is the nuchal translucency (NT), and this will be discussed in more detail later.

More recently other markers have been found to be useful in screening for trisomy 21 including the absence of the nasal bone, reversed a-wave in the ductus venosus and tricuspid regurgitation, and increased flow in the fetal hepatic artery. These markers when used with the combined test can increase the detection rate from 85–95% to 93–96% with a reduction of false positives from 5% to 2.5%.

NT is a measure of the maximum thickness of the translucent space in the tissue behind the fetal neck. It is a normal feature of the developing fetus and its thickness normally increases with CRL. Measurements are typically taken between 11 and 13^{+6} weeks when the CRL is between 45 and 84 mm and the space behind the neck is clearly translucent. Transabdominal USS is the preferred modality, but if views are suboptimal TVS is used.

Increase in this space may be a result of subcutaneous edema, altered composition of the extracellular fluid, abnormal development of the lymphatic system, or drainage failure of the lymphatic system. Conditions leading to these defects include cardiac failure, neuromuscular disorders, anemia, hypoproteinemia, congenital infection, diaphragmatic hernia, and skeletal dysplasia. Extensive studies have shown an association between many of these conditions and chromosomal abnormalities.

With increasing thickness there is a greater association with fetal abnormality. In the routine screening population NT measurement >3 mm has a sensitivity of 70% for all aneuploidy and 62% for trisomy 21 with a 4% false positive rate. However, use of a single cutoff to define thickness is inappropriate due to the effect of increasing gestational age. Therefore, use of the 95th percentile for a particular gestational age as a cutoff in combination with CRL is recommended.

Biochemical markers PAPP-A and free βhCG are included in the combined test. The inclusion of biochemical parameters adds an additional 16% to the detection rate obtained compared with NT and maternal age alone.

The absence of the nasal bone has a strong association with trisomy 21, 18, and 13. There is a higher incidence with increasing NT thickness. It also has a higher incidence in normal Afro-Caribbean babies when compared to Caucasians, and so when used to calculate risk, parental ethnic origin needs to be taken into account.

There is a higher risk of aneuploidy in multifetal pregnancies and a high false positive rate in first trimester screening. Risk is calculated per pregnancy in monochorionic pregnancies and for each baby in diamniotic and higher order nonidentical pregnancies. For triplet pregnancies, it is recommended that only NT and maternal age is used to assess risk.

Miscarriage rates are also increased with increasing nuchal thickness and are in keeping with the high association with chromosomal abnormalities. If positive screening leads to more invasive testing using amniocentesis or chorionic villus sampling (CVS), the risk of miscarriage is increased further and needs to be taken into account when counseling older women in the RPL clinic.

> **PATIENT ADVICE**
>
> Women who have experienced RPL may be reluctant to report subsequent pregnancies early for fear of repeat miscarriage. However, this should be discouraged as supportive care can be offered in early pregnancy and this has good outcome for couples with idiopathic RPL. Also first trimester screening for aneuploidy using the combined test is more accurate than using just serum tests in the second trimester.

Second trimester screening

RPL in the first trimester is generally not associated with a significant increase in the risk of second trimester miscarriage; however, some women will also give a history of second trimester loss. The role of cervical length assessments in women with a history of second trimester loss and preterm labor is well established, although in many of these cases, the cause is multifactorial, with a significant number being related to infection and chorioamnionitis with or without cervical weakness.

Screening for the risk of preterm delivery is now being offered in the form of cervical length assessment at the routine anomaly scan in many centers. This is typically performed between 20 and 24 weeks. The routine use of cervical length surveillance in other groups such as asymptomatic women and those with other risk factors such as recurrent early pregnancy loss, excisional treatment to the cervix, and congenital uterine anomalies is not so clear. There is evidence for using cervical cerclage in reducing births before 33 weeks in women with a history of mid-trimester loss and/or preterm delivery found to have a cervical length <25 mm before 24 weeks. Asymptomatic women with a history of three or more preterm deliveries and/or mid-trimester loss have been shown to benefit from prophylactic cervical cerclage between 12 and 14 weeks without prior ultrasound assessment of cervical length.

There are no specific studies looking at the role of cervical length assessment in women with recurrent early pregnancy loss. However, in the absence of effective treatment and limited guidance on the frequency of examinations, the routine use of cervical length assessment in women with recurrent early pregnancy loss is yet to be established. In addition, the lack of evidence to support the role of cervical cerclage, outside of the aforementioned indications, in women with a short cervix makes management unclear in this group.

Progesterone to prevent pregnancy loss

A large multicenter trial of 24 620 attending for routine anomaly scans found 1.7% of the women to have cervical length of ≤15 mm. The use of progesterone between 24 and 34 weeks reduced the risk of preterm birth in this group. A few small studies have shown that supplementation with progesterone in the first trimester can improve pregnancy outcome in subsequent pregnancies of women with a history of RPL. The results of a multicenter double blind RCT: the "Progesterone in Recurrent Miscarriage (PROMISE) Study" is awaited (ISRCTN92644181). This trial aims to answer this question and is currently recruiting.

Further assessment

A few studies have shown that there may be an increased risk of low birth weight babies and preterm delivery in subsequent pregnancies of women with a history of RPL. One suggestion for this is that it is a familial trait as another study has reported that women with RPL themselves had a higher incidence of preterm delivery and low birth weight at birth, compared to controls. This association may also be related to increased maternal age. Serial growth scans are not yet routinely used for women with idiopathic RPL but should be considered especially in women with other risk factors such as a previous low birth weight baby.

Supportive care

EPUs have developed with the aim of providing a one-stop outpatient service to women with abdominal pain, vaginal bleeding, or anxiety in early pregnancy. Supportive care has been variably described as open access to a dedicated specialist nurse in an EPU and to serial scanning throughout the first trimester. It has been suggested that the outcome of subsequent pregnancies in women with a history of unexplained recurrent first trimester pregnancy loss may be improved by supportive care. It has also been suggested that the pregnancy success rate may be improved in women who receive specific antenatal counseling and psychological support. The mechanism for this possible benefit is unclear; however, it is likely to reduce anxiety levels and the evidence can be used to reassure women who request empirical drug intervention.

Supportive care is recommended during the next pregnancy for women with unexplained RPL in the current guidelines from the European Society of Human Reproduction and Embryology (ESHRE) and the RCOG.

Table 10.1 Preferred Supportive Care Options for Women with Unexplained RM During Next Pregnancy ($n = 15$)

Domain 1: Medical Supportive Care	Domain 2: Nonmedical Supportive Care	Domain 3: Other Types of Supportive Care
Make a plan for the first 12 weeks with their gynecologist	From gynecologist	Women prefer an increase in partner involvement
Receive advice from their gynecologist concerning life style, diet and internet sites	Enquire how the patient is doing and what her emotional needs are	The need for supportive care directly after a miscarriage
Preference of one or max two well-informed gynecologists	Take the women seriously	Feel unhappy in the waiting room with visibly pregnant women
Receive frequent ultrasounds in early pregnancy and during symptoms	Give the women the feeling they are listened to and understood	
ßHCG blood monitoring before first ultrasound	Counseling from social worker	
Receive medication only if it is safe for the child	Experiencing supportive care from family, friends, and peer groups	
	Relaxation tools to unwind	
	Bereavement therapy for patients and explanation of bereavement levels for gynecologists	

Reproduced with Permission from Oxford University Press, Musters AM, Taminiau-Bloem E, van den Boogaard E *et al*. Supportive care for women with unexplained recurrent miscarriage: patient' perspectives. *Human Reproduction* 2011; 26: 873–877.

The type of supportive care preferred by women with idiopathic RPL has been assessed and can be seen in Table 10.1. Much of the preferred care centers around communication, counseling, and planning during early pregnancy in addition to serial ultrasound scans. The exact frequency of scans is unclear and the authors recommend fortnightly scans from 6 weeks gestation in the absence of symptoms and easy access to specialist nurses by telephone or in person. The ability to provide such a service carries staffing, training, and cost implications, and each unit will need to determine the level of supportive care that can be provided.

Conclusion

The role of assessment and monitoring of pregnancies at increased risk of miscarriage in the first trimester remains unclear. Although serum markers such as serum progesterone and serum βhCG are frequently used in clinical practice to monitor early pregnancies, they have been found to be more useful in assessing ectopic and PUL, rather than being able to predict miscarriage.

With the availability of TVS in dedicated EPUs, pregnancies can be diagnosed earlier, resulting in an inevitable increase in the incidence of PUL. The ideal gestation for performing the first scan is probably around 6 weeks in order to guarantee visualization of a normally developing pregnancy. Caution should be exercised when diagnosing miscarriage in early pregnancy and a repeat scan should be performed if there is any uncertainty. Supportive care alone remains the mainstay of the management of women with idiopathic RPL.

Bibliography

Nicolaides K 2011 Screening for fetal aneuploidies at 11 to 13 weeks. Prenatal Diagnosis; 31:7–15.

Oppenraaij, R. Jauniaux, E. Christiansen, O. Horcajadas, J. Farquharson, R. and Exalto N. Predicting adverse obstetric outcome after early pregnancy events and complications: a review. Human Reproduction Update (2009) **15** (4), 409–421.

Royal College of Obstetricians and Gynaecologists (RCOG) (2011) The Investigation and Treatment of Couples with Recurrent First-trimester and Second trimester Miscarriage. Green-top Guideline No. 17. RCOG Press, London.

11

Obstetric Complications in Patients with Recurrent Miscarriage – How Should they be Monitored in the Third Trimester?

Shehnaaz Jivraj[1,2]

[1] Jessop Wing, Sheffield Teaching Hospitals Trust, Sheffield, UK
[2] University of Sheffield, Sheffield, UK

Introduction

Miscarriage has been described to represent only the tip of the ice-berg of the amount of reproductive wastage that actually does happen. Historical reports have stated that out of 1000 conceptuses, only 728 make it to the implantation stage and out of these, 568 reach the stage of being clinically recognized as pregnancy, with 514 making it to the fetal stage. The rate of fetal loss then declines and only 500 result in a live-birth.

The pathology that underpins this spectrum of adverse pregnancy outcome may manifest itself as failed implantation, miscarriage, or later pregnancy complications such as intrauterine growth restriction (IUGR), preeclampsia, preterm delivery, or still birth. For this reason, women who have recurrent miscarriage are at a risk of later pregnancy complications as well, and this is supported by findings in epidemiological studies.

Traditionally, the causes of recurrent miscarriage have been divided into the following categories:

- chromosomal
- endocrine
- anatomical
- immunological
- prothrombotic
- unexplained (idiopathic)

This chapter will focus on the third trimester of pregnancy management of women with recurrent miscarriage who have been included in one of the aforementioned categories. However, investigations available in the third trimester to prevent adverse outcome followed by obstetric risks associated with various causes of recurrent miscarriage will first be discussed.

Recurrent Pregnancy Loss, First Edition. Edited by Ole B. Christiansen.
© 2014 John Wiley & Sons, Ltd. Published 2014 by John Wiley & Sons, Ltd.

Tests of fetal well-being in the third trimester – what are they and what do they mean

Ancillary tests of fetal well-being in the third trimester include the following:
    Noninvasive tests:

1. maternal subjective assessment of fetal movements
2. clinical examination of symphysial-fundal height
3. cardiotocography (CTG)
4. ultrasound scan (USS) for measurement of fetal growth and amniotic fluid index (AFI)
5. Doppler blood flow in the umbilical artery, middle cerebral artery, and ductus venosus
6. biophysical profile (BPP)

While clinical examination has its use, CTG and USS provide more objective parameters of fetal well-being.

CTGs are interpreted using the four basic parameters baseline rate, variability, the presence of accelerations and decelerations. Automated CTG measurements using Dawes–Redman criteria offer a more standardized computerized facility which also includes short term variation in the analysis.

Umbilical artery Doppler waveforms are used to measure the resistance and pulsatility indices using measurements of blood flow during fetal systole and diastole, retrograde flow in the ductus venosus denoted by an "a" wave resulting from atrial contraction, and the peak systolic velocity in the middle cerebral artery.

BPP is a scoring system using five criteria (Manning criteria), each scoring either zero or two points depending on whether the criterion is met or not. The scores are added together. The highest score possible is 10. A score of 8–10 predicts a perinatal mortality risk of less than 1 per 1000 in the ensuing week while a score of 0 predicts a perinatal mortality risk of 600 per 1000. The Manning criteria are shown in Table 11.1.

The purpose of all these tests of fetal well-being is to detect fetal growth restriction and the fetus at risk of intrauterine fetal death (IUFD) due to utero-placental insufficiency. This provides an opportunity to administer steroids to enhance fetal lung maturity, and plan a timely delivery by induction of labor or Caesarean section.

Table 11.1 Manning Criteria Used for BPP

	2	0
Reactive CTG	≥2 accelerations of 15 beats per min for 15 s in 30 min	<2 accelerations in 30 min
Fetal breathing movement	30 s sustained fetal breathing movements	Not sustained
Fetal movements	≥3 movements in 30 min	<3 movements in 30 min
Fetal tone	At least one flexion to extension and back	No flexion/extension
Amniotic fluid	2 cm depth in two perpendicular planes	<2 cm pocket

Prediction of spontaneous preterm labor

The accurate prediction of preterm delivery is notoriously difficult. A combination of cervical length assessment and fetal fibronectin (fFN) is clinically employed to identify both symptomatic and asymptomatic women at risk of preterm delivery. fFN appears to have an excellent negative predictive value and thus offers the ability to facilitate decision making regarding tocolysis, administration of corticosteroids and arranging in-utero transfer to facilities with neonatal intensive care.

Prevention of adverse effects of prematurity

Antenatal corticosteroids administered before preterm delivery reduces the risk of cerebroventricular hemorrhage, necrotizing enterocolitis, and systemic infections by up to 50% and requirement for respiratory support and intensive care admissions by up to 20% in the first 48 h of life. A single course of antenatal corticosteroids should be considered routine for preterm delivery with few exceptions. One recommended regime is a single course of Betamethasone 12 mg given intramuscularly as two doses over 24 h.

Repeat doses of corticosteroids are not routinely recommended.

If preterm labor ensues, in the absence of contraindications, tocolytics such as atosiban should be administered. This is done primarily for the purpose of buying time to administer corticosteroids and if indicated, transfer of the patient for delivery to a unit which has neonatal intensive care facilities.

Management of preterm prelabor rupture of membranes (PPROM)

PPROM is a common precursor of preterm birth. PPROM may occur as a result of subclinical genital tract infection. In the United Kingdom, the results of the ORACLE trial form the basis of the use of prophylactic antibiotics in the management of PPROM. The ORACLE trial was a randomized placebo controlled trial of Erythromycin versus Co-amoxiclav in women who present with PPROM. Use of erythromycin was associated with prolongation of pregnancy, reduction in neonatal treatment with surfactant, decrease in oxygen dependence at 28 days of age and older, fewer major cerebral abnormalities on ultrasonography before discharge, and fewer positive blood cultures. Co-amoxiclav was associated with a significantly higher rate of neonatal necrotizing enterocolitis. Benefits of antibiotic usage were not seen when women presented with preterm labor with intact membranes.

Our own practice is to administer Erythromycin 250 mg four times daily for 10 days or until delivery if this occurs sooner. This is in addition to administering cortico-steroids to promote fetal lung maturity. Cervical and vaginal swabs are done together with a screen for Group B streptococcus colonization. This generally includes a rectal swab as well. If labor does not start spontaneously after 48 h, the patient is monitored as an outpatient with admission for delivery if there are signs of infection. The woman monitors the color of her amniotic fluid, her own temperature, and attends for twice weekly CTGs and weekly USS for umbilical artery Doppler measurements. In the absence of fetal compromise or clinical infection, labor is induced at 36 completed weeks, although at present there is an argument for inducing labor at 34 completed weeks, as the risk of chorioamnionitis after 34 weeks may outweigh the benefit of waiting for fetal lung maturity.

Routine use of prophylactic antibiotics for preterm labor with intact membranes in the absence of clinically proven infection is not recommended.

Management of third trimester pregnancy in diagnostic categories of recurrent miscarriage

Chromosomal Abnormalities

Parental chromosomal abnormalities are found in 3–5% of couples presenting to any recurrent miscarriage clinic. The most common abnormality is a balanced transloca-tion and the female partner is twice as likely to be affected as the male partner. When such an abnormality is discovered at initial screening, couples are referred for genetic counseling. The likely outcomes in a future pregnancy are miscarriage of a normal fetus (sporadic miscarriage), miscarriage of fetus of abnormal karyotype, live birth of a normal child, or rarely live birth of an affected child with an unbalanced trans-location and resultant multiple congenital abnormalities and learning difficulties. Genetic counseling serves to provide information in the likelihood of the outcome based on the type of abnormality. Women should be offered prenatal diagnosis. In the case of an unaffected pregnancy, no further action needs to be taken other than routine antenatal care. If an affected pregnancy goes past viability, antenatal care will need to be more tailored. In one particular observational study, out of 278 carrier couples, two affected pregnancies were discovered at prenatal diagnosis and were subsequently terminated and there were two live-births of affected offspring. In this particular study, after a mean follow-up period of 5.8 years, the miscarriage rate was higher in carrier couples (49 vs. 30%), but the eventual live-birth rate of an unaffected child was similar in the two groups (83 vs. 84%).

If pregnancy has been a result of in vitro fertilization and preimplantation genetic screening (IVF-PGS), such a pregnancy should be considered for increased surveil-lance by virtue of IVF being a risk factor for IUGR and preeclampsia.

An ongoing pregnancy affected by a chromosomal abnormality would be at risk of severe IUGR and still birth. From 28 weeks gestation onwards, growth scans should be undertaken together with ancillary tests of fetal well-being, namely, liquor volume, Doppler measurements, and CTGs. Steroids should be administered if delivery is likely before 36 weeks. A pediatric alert should be made antenatally and often parents may find it helpful to have discussed anticipated management of an affected child with a pediatrician in advance of delivery.

In case of anticipated surgery after birth, delivery may need to be planned in a setup with pediatric surgical facilities.

Endocrine disorders

Thyroid Hormone Disorders

An increased quantity of circulating estradiol in pregnancy stimulates hepatic expression of thyroxine binding globulin (TBG). There is thus a twofold increase in circulating TBG. The excess TBG mops up free circulating thyroxine, lowering circulating thyroxine levels. The existing feedback loop stimulates an increase in thyroid stimulating hormone (TSH) production by the pituitary gland resulting in an increase in thyroxine production by the thyroid gland. Further, human chorionic gonadotropin (hCG), which is structurally similar to TSH also stimulates the thyroid gland. The net effect is a renewed equilibrium between free and bound thyroid hormones with an increase in total T3 and T4. An increased glomerular filtration rate increases iodide clearance by the kidneys. There is also increased iodide uptake by the developing fetus. The result is an increased demand for iodine in pregnancy.

Pathology

An increased demand on the thyroid gland is reached by 20 weeks and stays elevated until term. In normal healthy women, this increased load on the thyroid gland is not a burden but in subclinical hypothyroidism, the extra demand on the thyroid gland can precipitate disease. If pregnancy ensues, associated complications are raised blood pressure, lowered IQ, physical and mental retardation (cretinism), and IUFD. The associated risks of hyperthyroidism are preeclampsia, preterm labor, low birth weight, and fetal and perinatal death. It has been hypothesized that thyroid autoantibodies, in euthyroid women, may cause thyroid damage but the thyroid gland sufficiently compensates in the nonpregnant state. In pregnancy, this effort to compensate may be sufficient to keep a woman euthyroid biochemically, but not clinically. Thus thyroid function tests (TFTs) may show alteration reflecting a strain on the thyroid gland but the T3, T4, and TSH values may remain within normal laboratory reference ranges. Normal ranges in a laboratory usually represent values from 95 to 99% of the population. T3, T4, and TSH laboratory values are not calculated separately for individuals with antithyroid antibodies.

Antithyroid Antibodies

Antithyroid antibodies are present in 10–20% of the population of reproductive age group. The antibody that has been associated with poor reproductive outcome in euthyroid women is thyroid peroxidase antibody (TPOAb). A recent meta-analysis of case–control and cohort studies by Thangaratinam *et al.* (2011) found a higher miscarriage rate in carriers of thyroid autoantibodies in the recurrent miscarriage population (OR 4.22; 95% CI 0.97–18.44) and in the subfertile population (OR 3.15; 95% CI 2.23–4.44) compared with noncarriers. Compared with women without thyroid antibodies, women with thyroid autoantibodies had higher TSH levels (OR 0.51; 95% CI 0.14–0.88), suggesting an increase in the demand for thyroxine synthesis. The risk of preterm birth was doubled among carriers of the antibodies (OR 2.07; 95% CI 1.17–3.68) compared with noncarriers. This observation begs the question – should women with thyroid antibodies be given thyroxine supplementation? Two small randomized studies showed a lower miscarriage rate in euthyroid women with thyroid autoantibodies given thyroxine. Among women with recurrent miscarriage and thyroid autoantibodies, a randomized controlled trial (TABLET trial) is currently underway in the United Kingdom to determine if supplementation with levothyroxine increases the proportion of women who attain a live birth beyond 34 completed weeks and survival at 28 days of neonatal life.

It is recommended that women with thyroid autoantibodies have monthly TFTs during pregnancy, have USSs to check for IUGR from 28 weeks onwards, and be warned of symptoms of preterm labor. Women who are likely to need delivery before 36 weeks because of IUGR or women who present in preterm labor should be given a course of steroids to enhance fetal lung maturity.

Polycystic Ovary Syndrome (PCOS)

In 2004, the Rotterdam criteria were established to define PCOS. These consisted of two out of the following three criteria:

1. oligo/anovulation or oligo/amenorrhea
2. clinical or biochemical hyperandrogenism
3. polycystic ovaries

The reported incidence of PCOS in women of reproductive age is 3–15% depending on the population studied and the diagnostic criteria used to define PCOS. Of the women with recurrent miscarriage 40% have polycystic ovaries but if the Rotterdam criteria are used, PCOS is found in 8–10% of women with recurrent miscarriage. A recent large Swedish population based cohort study that compared pregnancy outcomes among 3787 births in women with PCOS and 1 191 336 births among women without PCOS reported an increased risk of gestational diabetes (RR 2.32; 95% CI 1.88–2.88), preeclampsia (RR 1.45; 95% CI 1.24–1.69), very preterm birth defined as birth <32 weeks gestation (RR 2.21; 95% CI 1.69–2.90), meconium aspiration (RR 2.02; 95% CI 1.13–3.61), Caesarean section (RR 1.18; 95% CI 1.07–1.29), Apgar scores <7 at 5 min (RR 1.41; 95% CI 1.09–1.83), and large for gestational age babies (RR 1.39; 95% CI 1.19–1.62). Larger prospective studies are needed to elucidate which components of PCOS may be predictive of specific complications such as gestational diabetes or preeclampsia as it may well be that it is obesity rather than other components of PCOS that is the risk factor for the perinatal complications seen in PCOS patients. Until the clinical implications of this broad condition are made clearer, women should be considered at increased risk of perinatal complications, should be monitored appropriately with delivery in hospital and specifically in a unit with neonatal care facilities. Such women should therefore have a glucose tolerance test between 24 and 28 weeks and subsequently be monitored for IUGR throughout the remainder of the third trimester.

Structural Uterine Abnormalities

Embryologically, the uterus forms by fusion of the paramesonephric ducts. Incomplete fusion or failure of resorption of the intervening septum can result in a spectrum of abnormalities ranging from a uterus didelphys to a bicornuate uterus to the presence of a uterine septum to a unicornuate uterus. Out of all these abnormalities, the one associated with recurrent miscarriage most strongly is the uterine septum.

The presence of a uterine septum is associated with an increased risk of preterm delivery. Still birth has also been reported to be associated with the presence of a uterine septum. Resection of the septum has been shown to reduce both preterm delivery and still birth rate in retrospective studies but the risk is not eliminated altogether. A recent systematic review which classified all canalization defects into a single group showed a preterm birth rate which was twice as high as normal controls (RR 2.14; 95% CI 1.48–3.11). The exact mechanism of this association is not known but it has been suggested that the endometrium overlying a septum is abnormal and results in poor implantation resulting in a spectrum of adverse outcome. It has also been suggested that the presence of an anatomical abnormality results in distortion of the uterine cavity with a reduced capacity and higher propensity for onset of preterm labor. It is not possible to prevent the onset of preterm labor in this group of women. However, should preterm labor ensue, tocolytics should be used appropriately to allow time for administration of steroids to enhance fetal lung maturity. As these women are at risk of malpresentation, it is advisable that such women have a presentation check by USS at 36 weeks gestation or if labor starts spontaneously. The absence of a presenting part in the pelvis carries a risk of umbilical cord prolapse should membranes rupture spontaneously.

Fibroids
Fibroids are classified into submucous, intramural or subserous by their location. Submucous fibroids are further divided into type 0, I, II fibroids depending on the extent of myometrial extension. They are present in 8–10% of women with recurrent miscarriage and removal is recommended for those fibroids that distort the endometrial cavity. Fibroids that distort the endometrial cavity are usually suitable for hysteroscopic resection. Sometimes, fibroids may be resected via laparotomy or laparoscopy. In these circumstances as long as the endometrial cavity is not breached, risk of uterine rupture is not increased and patients may have a vaginal delivery. If the endometrial cavity is entered at the time of surgical excision, such that the full thickness of the uterus has been breached, then such a patient would need a Caesarean section for delivery because of the associated risk of uterine scar rupture. The exact magnitude of the risk of uterine rupture, however, remains uncertain.

Large fibroids >5 cm in diameter have been associated with a higher preterm delivery rate than smaller fibroids or no fibroids. Large fibroids are also associated with more blood loss at delivery and a greater need for postpartum blood transfusion than in cases of smaller fibroids or no fibroids. The underlying mechanism for this remains unclear. It has been suggested that an abnormal immune, metabolic or vascular milieu in the region of the fibroid may impair implantation and the anatomical distortion caused may decrease uterine distensibility and uterine contractility.

Ashermann's Syndrome
Ashermann's syndrome is a rare cause of recurrent miscarriage. It occurs as a complication of endometritis or overzealous curettage, resulting in the loss of the basal layer of the endometrium. It can result in implantation failure. However if pregnancy does ensue, or if pregnancy occurs after treatment, for the condition there is a risk of morbidly adherent placenta of varying degrees. It is helpful to detect this antenatally and plan delivery. Delivery carries a risk of retained placenta, postpartum hemorrhage and hysterectomy. The risk of a morbidly adherent placenta occurs with any uterine scarring including previous myomectomy and Caesarean section.

Antenatal ultrasound may help to detect this. Features include the presence of placental lacunae, obliteration of the clear space between the placenta and the uterus, interruption of the bladder border, a lower uterine segment thickness of less than 1 mm in case of a previous Caesarean section and Doppler flow characteristics. If suspected, MRI scanning can further assist diagnosis.

Prothrombotic conditions

Primary Antiphospholipid Syndrome

A diagnosis of the primary antiphospholipid syndrome is made on the basis of one or more clinical criteria together with the presence of lupus anticoagulant or elevated levels of anticardiolipin or anti B2 glycoprotein 1 antibodies taken on two occasions at least 12 weeks apart. The obstetric criteria for diagnosis are as follows:

1. three first trimester miscarriages
2. one miscarriage after 10 weeks gestation of a morphologically normal fetus
3. preterm delivery <34 weeks gestation due to IUGR or preeclampsia

Treatment consists of a combination of low dose aspirin and low molecular weight heparin from the diagnosis of pregnancy until at least 34 weeks gestation. Some of these women may require thromboprophylaxis throughout pregnancy and in the postpartum period, depending on the presence of other risk factors for VTE.

Without treatment such women have a live-birth rate of 10–40% depending on the type of antiphospholipid antibody present and the cutoff titers used to make the diagnosis, which improves to 70% when treated with aspirin and low molecular weight heparin. Despite treatment, women are at risk of increased obstetric complications. In one particular study of 150 women with the primary antiphospholipid syndrome treated with aspirin and low molecular weight heparin, 71% resulted in a live birth. Forty-one pregnancies (27%) miscarried, the majority in the first trimester. One woman delivered a still birth baby, and one a premature baby who died in the neonatal period. One pregnancy was terminated for a fetal anomaly. Gestational hypertension complicated 17% of pregnancies. Twenty-six babies (24%) were delivered before 37 weeks of gestation. Fifty women (46%) were delivered by caesarean section. The median birth weight of all live born infants was 3069 g (range 531–4300). Of the infants, 15% (16/108) were small for gestational age (SGA).

Doppler assessment of the uterine arteries between 16–18 weeks and 22–24 weeks has been used to select out those women with the primary antiphospholipid syndrome at risk of preeclampsia and SGA. The presence of bilateral uterine artery notching at 22–24 weeks was found to be predictive of preeclampsia and SGA only in women with lupus anticoagulant (45 out of 170 women had lupus anticoagulant). In predicting preeclampsia, bilateral uterine artery notching at 22–24 weeks showed a positive predictive value of 75% and a negative predictive value of 94%. In predicting SGA, bilateral uterine artery notching at 22–24 weeks had a positive predictive value of 80% and a negative predictive value of 94%. Uterine artery Doppler was however of limited value in predicting preeclampsia or SGA in pregnancies associated with anticardiolipin antibodies alone.

Historically, and based on histological studies of products of conception from women with antiphospholipid antibodies, the pathogenesis of antiphospholipid antibody related pregnancy loss was thought to be thrombotic. Recent histological studies and in vitro data have suggested that antiphospholipid antibody related pregnancy loss is the result of impaired trophoblast invasion and defective implantation, the effect of which is reversed by heparin.

Risks of Treatment

Heparin-induced thrombocytopenia (HIT) is a complication of heparin treatment caused by antibodies directed against complexes of platelet factor 4 and heparin. In one reported small series of 13 cases of HIT, low molecular weight heparin was the causative agent in eight (62%) patients. Immunological assays currently employed may lead to an over diagnosis of the condition. Fortunately, there have been few if any reported cases of HIT as a consequence of prophylactic dose administration of low molecular weight heparin in pregnancy. It is therefore recommended that a full blood count to monitor platelet levels in a woman on prophylactic doses of low molecular weight heparin should be done once a month and the frequency of monitoring increased together with involvement of a hematologist if the platelet count starts to drop.

Long term low molecular weight heparin therapy may be associated with osteoporosis. This was deemed to be one disadvantage of treatment particularly in areas where low molecular weight heparin is given without scientific evidence of benefit to pregnancy outcome. It must however be noted also that pregnancy itself as well as lactation causes a reduction in bone mineral density (BMD). Moreover, it has been reported that up to 8% of women are already osteopenic at the start of pregnancy. To determine whether heparin treatment worsens the loss in BMD that already occurs in pregnancy, a prospective study was carried out to compare T scores (a score which compares the BMD with a younger population) from the BMD measurement at the lumbar spine, the femoral neck, and forearm using dual energy x-ray absorptiometry (DEXA) scans. DEXA scans were carried out at 12 weeks gestation, immediately postpartum and at 12 weeks postpartum among 123 women who had the primary antiphospholipid syndrome treated with aspirin and heparin. 46 women took unfractionated heparin and 77 took low molecular weight heparin. During pregnancy, BMD decreased by 3.7% ($P < 0.001$) at the lumbar spine and by 0.9% ($P < 0.05$) at the neck of femur with no significant change at the forearm. Lactation was associated with a significant decrease in the lumbar spine and neck of femur BMD. There was no significant difference in BMD changes between the two heparin preparations. There was no control group of untreated women in this study for comparison, but the authors reported that the reduction in BMD observed in their study was similar to the reduction reported in untreated pregnancies. Based on this data of a relevant population (recurrent miscarriage and antiphospholipid syndrome) women may be reassured that the loss in BMD that occurs with prophylactic doses of low molecular weight heparin used to treat this condition in pregnancy is no greater than that which occurs in a normal pregnancy. It is not recommended that women should have any additional BMD tests to check for osteopenia or osteoporosis routinely before starting or after completion of treatment for recurrent miscarriage associated primary anti-phospholipid syndrome.

If a woman on aspirin and heparin presents with vaginal bleeding, a platelet count should be determined to rule out HIT and an obstetric cause for her vaginal bleeding sought on history and examination. Vaginal bleeding per se should not be a reason to stop treatment.

☆ TIPS AND TRICKS

The primary antiphospholipid syndrome should be diagnosed using a combination of clinical and laboratory criteria. Laboratory criteria consist of medium or high titer IgG or IgM anticardiolipin antibodies (>40GPL or >40MPL) or high titer antiB2GP1 antibodies (>99th percentile) or the presence of lupus anticoagulant.

Tests for antiphospholipid antibodies should be done at least 12 weeks after the clinical event and no later than 5 years after the event. A test done less than 12 weeks after the clinical event risks interference from the effects of the clinical event itself. A test done more than 5 years after the clinical event could raise doubt on the association of a result remote from the clinical event. A test of confirmation should be done at least 12 weeks after the first test.

Anti Ro/SS-A and Anti La/SS-B Antibodies

The secondary antiphospholipid syndrome refers to the presence of antiphospholipid antibodies in the presence of systemic lupus erythematosus (SLE). Anti Ro/SS-A and anti La/SS-B antibodies are strongly associated with connective tissue disorders such as SLE. Note that 1–2% of offspring of women with anti Ro/SS-A antibodies have congenital heart block. It has been recommended that in women with anti Ro/SS-A antibodies serial fetal cardiac and obstetric ultrasound is performed from 16 weeks onwards to detect signs of early fetal abnormalities, such as premature atrial contractions or pericardial effusion, that might precede complete atrioventricular block and that might be a target of preventive therapy.

Inherited thrombophilia

The most common inherited thrombophilia among Caucasians is factor V Leiden. The reported allele frequency of this mutation is similar between women with recurrent miscarriage and the general obstetric population at approximately 4%. However, among women with recurrent miscarriage, the risk of a further miscarriage is higher among carriers of factor V Leiden than among women with unexplained recurrent miscarriage. Consequently, many clinicians choose to offer low dose low molecular weight heparin to these women on an empirical basis in the hope of improving live-birth rate. It has to be noted, however, that there are no data in the form of any randomized controlled trial to suggest that treating women with factor V

Leiden and recurrent miscarriage actually improves pregnancy outcome. Often, as part of routine investigations for recurrent miscarriage, other thrombophilia are screened for, namely, antithrombin III, protein C and protein S deficiency and prothrombin G20210A. The British Society for Haematology recommends that antithrombotic therapy should not be given to pregnant women based on heritable tests for thrombophilia with the aim of improving pregnancy outcome. An inadvertently detected thrombophilia however may add to the venous-thromboembolism (VTE) risk of the pregnant woman and under these circumstances, it may be necessary to plan postnatal thromboprophylaxis or indeed give antenatal thromboprophylaxis.

Other risk factors for VTE include a personal history of VTE, family history of VTE, significant active comorbidities such as heart or lung disease, SLE, inflammatory bowel disease, cancer, nephritic syndrome, myeloproliferative disorders, BMI >40, and immobility.

Based on guidance from the Department of Health (UK) and the Royal College of Obstetricians and Gynaecologists (UK), if there are three or more persisting risk factors, consideration should be given to continuing thromboprophylaxis throughout pregnancy and for 6 weeks postpartum.

While case–control studies and hence retrospective data have shown an association of heritable thrombophilia with IUGR and preeclampsia, routine administration of antenatal thromboprophylaxis has not been shown to reduce these risks. However based on retrospective data, it is advisable to monitor these women for both IUGR and preeclampsia from 28 weeks onwards.

✋ CAUTION

Testing for thrombophilia other than the primary antiphospholipid syndrome and factor V Leiden should not be undertaken routinely unless there are risk factors for thrombosis such as a personal or family history of VTE.

The British Society for Haematology (2010) suggests that therapeutic decisions for anticoagulant treatment should be based on clinical circumstances and not on the results of thrombophilia testing. Antithrombotic therapy should not be given to pregnant women based on tests for heritable thrombophilia to prevent obstetric complications. Randomized controlled trials with a placebo arm in women with pregnancy complications and heritable thrombophilia are in place, and if these studies indicate a benefit of treatment only then would there be a rationale for thrombophilia testing and treatment.

PEARLS TO TAKE HOME

Aspirin and heparin are proven treatment for the primary antiphospholipid syndrome. Despite treatment, these women remain at risk of later pregnancy complications such as preeclampsia and IUGR.

If a thrombophilia is inadvertently discovered, look for other risk factors for thrombosis in pregnancy before withholding or planning thromboprophylaxis.

Table 11.2 Obstetric Complications Associated with Recurrent Miscarriage as a Group (All Causes Including Unexplained Recurrent Miscarriage)

	Cases n = 162 (%)	Controls n = 24 699 (%)	Significance
Diabetes	1.7	0.8	$0.1 < P < 0.15$
Hypertension	7.3	11	$0.15 < P < 0.2$
Preterm delivery	13.3	4	$P < 0.001$
SGA	13	2	$P < 0.01$
Perinatal mortality	2.5	1	$P < 0.05$
Caesarean section	36	16	$P < 0.001$
Instrumental delivery	14	17	$0.3 < P < 0.4$

Unexplained recurrent miscarriage

The current recommendation for treatment of women with unexplained recurrent miscarriage is supportive care in the first trimester. This has been shown in observational studies to improve live-birth rate compared with routine antenatal care. Aspirin and low molecular weight heparin do not offer any additional benefit to this group of women. As a group, women with recurrent miscarriage are at risk of later pregnancy complications. Data from our own unit have shown a higher risk of obstetric and perinatal complications compared to the general obstetric population (Table 11.2). It must be stressed that these data refer to *all* women with recurrent miscarriage – including women with a diagnosis of *unexplained* recurrent miscarriage – and do not refer exclusively to women with unexplained recurrent miscarriage. It is therefore recommended that women with unexplained recurrent miscarriage as well are cared for in an obstetric unit that has facilities for perinatal/neonatal care.

PATIENT/PARENT ADVICE

Supportive care has been shown to improve pregnancy outcome when offered to women in the first trimester. While this support may be extended into the second and third trimester of pregnancy, women should be reassured that once a pregnancy safely crosses the threshold of 12 weeks, there is a high likelihood of a healthy live birth. This reassurance may take the form of shared care between her community midwife and her obstetrician so as to restore as much normality as possible in her daily activities. However, as pregnancy can be a highly stressful event for many of these women, with many women already suffering from underlying psychological disturbances, involvement of specialists in the field of maternal mental health should be undertaken sooner rather than later where indicated.

Multidisciplinary involvement is the key to modern and safer practice. Other disciplines to involve in a patient's care include maternal mental health, hematology, anesthetics, and neonatology.

Bibliography

Regan, L., Backos, M., Rai, R. (2011) The investigation and treatment of couples with recurrent miscarriage. Green-Top Guideline No. 17. Royal College of Obstetricians and Gynaecologists.

Jivraj, S. and Li, T.C. (2010) Thrombophilia, recurrent miscarriage and late pregnancy loss. *Journal of Paediatrics, Obstetrics & Gynaecology.* 213–220.

Miyakis, S., Lockshin, M.D., Atsumi, T. *et al.* (2006) International consensus statement on an update of the classification criteria for definite antiphospholipid syndrome (APS). *Journal of Thrombosis Haemostasis*, 4 (2), 295–306.

Thangaratinam S, Tan A, Knox E, Kilby MD, Franklyn J, Coomarasamy A. Association between thyroid autoantibodies and miscarriage and preterm birth: meta-analysis of evidence BMJ 2011;342:d2616.

12

Recurrent Miscarriage after ART: A Double Challenge

Elisabeth C. Larsen[1] and Ole B. Christiansen[1,2]

[1]Unit for Recurrent Miscarriage, Fertility Clinic 4071, Rigshospitalet, Copenhagen, Denmark
[2]Department of Obstetrics and Gynaecology, Aalborg University Hospital, Aalborg, Denmark

Introduction

In our clinic, approximately 35% of the RM patients at the time of referral are also undergoing ART defined as treatment with ovulation induction (OI) with or without intrauterine insemination (IUI) or in vitro fertilization (IVF) or intracytoplasmatic sperm injection (ICSI). The combination of RM and subfertility has in previous studies been shown to be associated with an increased risk of a further miscarriage. These patients have two problems to fight in their struggle to get a child, which renders the pressure on the medical staff for success in the next pregnancy even greater than in those with no concomitant infertility problems. Experiencing one or more miscarriages subsequent to ART after a long history of infertility is for many patients so emotionally overwhelming that they lose all hope to get a child and abandon further pregnancy attempts.

Two subsets of RM patients with a need for ART

Some of the RM patients in our clinic with a need for ART (group I) have originally had no problems to conceive but after a series of miscarriages they either completely fail to achieve conception or the time to pregnancy (TTP) had become so long that they seek ART. Other patients with combined ART and RM (group II) exhibit a history of primary infertility and have conceived by ART from the very beginning of their reproductive history but miscarried each time.

There are probably two main reasons for the courses in group I: (i) after a series of pregnancies ending in miscarriage many patients have entered the second part of the 30s – a period where TTP increases rapidly primarily due to diminished ovarian reserve and egg quality and (ii) each previous miscarriage whether surgically or medically treated poses a risk for tubal damage due to the risk of clinical and subclinical postabortem salpingitis. This is illustrated by findings in a recent study done in our clinic where RM patients in a questionnaire reported a 3% or 8% frequency of clinical pelvic inflammation after previous missed abortions treated surgically or medically, respectively.

Recurrent Pregnancy Loss, First Edition. Edited by Ole B. Christiansen.
© 2014 John Wiley & Sons, Ltd. Published 2014 by John Wiley & Sons, Ltd.

Table 12.1 Examples of Factors Suggested to Cause Clinical Miscarriage, Biochemical Pregnancies, or Both According to Presumed Causes of Infertility

OI with or without IUI		
Cause of Infertility	Cause of Miscarriages	Cause of Biochemical Pregnancies (PULs)
PCOS	High testosterone and LH. Obesity-related factors	High testosterone and LH. Obesity-related factors
Endometriosis	Inflammatory cytokines	Inflammatory cytokines. Tubal damage (ectopic pregnancies)
Male factor	DNA chromatin damage	DNA chromatin damage
Unexplained	Immunological factors Embryonal aneuploidy	Immunological factors Embryonal aneuploidy Tubal damage (ectopic pregnancies)

IVF/ICSI Treatment	
Cause of Infertility	Cause of Miscarriages or Biochemical Pregnancies
PCOS	High testosterone and LH. Obesity-related factors
Endometriosis	Inflammatory cytokines
Male factor	DNA chromatin damage
Tubal occlusion	Hydrosalpinx fluid leakage
Low ovarian reserve	Aneuploid eggs and embryos
Unexplained	Immunological factors. Embryonal aneuploidy
All causes	Method-related causes: Suppression of follicular phase LH High midcycle estrogen Excessive follicle stimulation Endometrial hyperstimulation In vitro culture

In group II, the possible causes for the co-occurrence of infertility and a RM diagnosis are summarized in Table 12.1. These putative causes should be considered separately in patients undergoing OI with or without IUI and in those undergoing IVF/ICSI. As shown in the upper part of Table 12.1, patients undergoing OI with or without IUI comprise a mixture of couples with ovulation abnormalities, endometriosis, subnormal sperm quality, or unexplained infertility. Some of these women have had genuine RM (miscarriages confirmed as intrauterine), whereas others present a history of mainly biochemical pregnancies (pregnancies of unknown location = PULs) and many of these may in fact be spontaneously resorbed ectopic pregnancies.

RM after OI with or without IUI

Women undergoing OI who have irregular ovulations most often have polycystic ovary syndrome (PCOS) and are often obese. PCOS may be directly associated with an increased risk of miscarriage due to high androgen or LH levels in the plasma and/or ovaries or the association may be indirect through the obesity. Obesity has been documented to be an independent risk factor for miscarriage, for example, in egg donation studies finding a 38% miscarriage rate in obese recipients of eggs from normal-weighted donors compared with a 13% miscarriage rate in normal-weight recipients. It is also possible that the increased miscarriage risk in PCOS patients may be related to the OI treatment that may result in ovulation and fertilization of aneuploid eggs, which would have low chance to be ovulated in nonstimulated cycles (see later in this chapter).

Some patients undergoing OI combined with IUI are subfertile due to documented or occult endometriosis. Endometriosis is often causing adhesions around the ovary and tubal ostium, increasing the risk of spontaneously resorbed ectopic pregnancies diagnosed as PULs but by the patients they are often reported as miscarriages. Endometriosis may also increase the risk of genuine miscarriage (although this is controversial) due to increased secretion of inflammatory cytokines in the pelvic peritoneum that may do harm to the eggs in the ovary or the embryos through the passage to the uterus. The postimplantation embryos may also be exposed to the inflammatory cytokines that have been transported from the pelvic endometrial lesions to the endometrium through the uterine veins.

Sperm-related factors may cause miscarriage after ART – this will be discussed later in the chapter.

Patients with unexplained infertility, who are offered treatment with OI combined with IUI, may comprise cases with normal passage of contrast by hysterosalpingography (HSG) but with occult tubal damage due to the lack of cilia or the presence of intratubal adhesions caused by previous pelvic inflammations. After OI with IUI, these patients will sometimes achieve clinical tubal pregnancy but often they will experience repeated PULs, which may result in a diagnosis of RM. In a study from our clinic it was found that in patients referred with the diagnosis of RM but who had a history of exclusively PULs and no miscarriages confirmed by ultrasound or histology, a very high rate(23.8%) of clinical ectopic pregnancies requiring surgery was found in the reproductive history. We therefore think that a subpopulation of patients with RM exists where the losses are due to recurrent spontaneously resorbed ectopic pregnancies.

RM after IVF/ICSI

The same endocrine and endometriosis-related and factors that can cause miscarriages after OI can probably also be risk factors for miscarriage after IVF/ICSI. In contrast to the situation after OI with or without IUI the risk of spontaneously resorbed ectopic pregnancies (being misclassified as miscarriages) after IVF/ICSI is low since the embryos are not going to pass through the tubes. Instead there will be other factors specific for the IVF/ICSI procedure that can increase the risk of miscarriage.

The infertility-causing factors that may increase the risk of miscarriage after IVF/ICSI include PCOS and endometriosis-related factors, as previously mentioned.

Some but not all relevant studies have suggested that sperm chromatin structure defects (detected in sperm chromatin structure assays = SCSAs) are associated with male factor infertility and poor outcome after IUI or IVF/ICSI. A meta-analysis of relevant studies found that elevated levels of sperm DNA damage were associated with a more than double risk of miscarriage after IVF/ICSI ($p < 0.00001$). One recent study found that 85% of male partners of couples with unexplained RM had a profile with high values of double-stranded DNA damage in the sperm compared with only 33% of fertile sperm donors, suggesting a specific paternal explanation in some of these couples.

Another factor that may increase the risk of miscarriage after IVF/ICSI is the presence of large sacto-/hydrosalpinges. In a meta-analysis of a series of relevant studies an early pregnancy loss rate of 44% was found in patients with hydrosalpinges undergoing IVF/ICSI compared with 31% in patients without hydrosalpinges. The mechanism may be fluid containing pro-inflammatory substances leaking from the hydrosalpinges into the uterine cavity, disturbing the implantation process.

It is clear that a diminished ovarian reserve as evidenced by a low antral follicle count at ultrasound examination, low levels of anti-Müllerian hormone, and a low number of aspirated eggs is an important cause of infertility and repeated implantation failure after IVF. The ovarian reserve decreases, and the risk of embryonal aneuploidy and thus miscarriage increases with age. However, it is more unclear whether the condition *diminished ovarian reserve per se* (which may be diagnosed even at a young age) is an independent predictor of miscarriage and RM. In several studies elucidating prognostic factors for live birth in women below 40 years of age and suffering from RM, maternal age was not a predictor of miscarriage after adjustment for other relevant independent risk factors. In addition, several studies have not been able to find that low levels of anti-Müllerian hormone in women with RM affect the prognosis for live birth after adjustment for age.

★ TIPS AND TRICKS

In patients of advanced age (>40 years), aneuploidy of eggs and thus also the embryos is the most likely cause of both infertility and RM after ART.

As discussed in Chapters 2, 3, and 4, several studies have suggested that a series of immunological abnormalities are found with increased prevalence in women with infertility, repeated implantation failure after IVF, and RM. High total NK cell numbers and CD56dim NK cells, a highTh1/Th2 cytokine ratio, the presence of a variety of autoantibodies (especially antiphospholipid and thyroid peroxydase antibodies) in the blood or the presence of specific polymorphisms in the maternal *HLA-G* gene may be risk factors for infertility, poor implantation rate after IVF/ICSI, and RM. Although much more and larger studies are needed to document the immunological link between the different conditions, if confirmed, this may be the basis for offering various forms of immunotherapy to patients with concomitant RM and ART treatment.

The procedures undertaken as part of IVF/ICSI procedures may cause an increased miscarriage rate, which has been reported to be increased independent of the cause of infertility.

The OI undertaken as part of IVF/ICSI procedures probably can cause ovulation of poor quality eggs that would not be ovulated in unstimulated cycles. This view is supported by a study showing that after IVF/ICSI with standard FSH stimulation and downregulation with gonadotropin releasing hormone (GnRH), the fraction of chromosomal abnormal embryos is increased compared with a mild stimulation protocol with the use of GnRH antagonists (73 vs. 55% embryos with aneuploidy, $p < 0.05$). Such aneuploid embryos are prone to be miscarried after transfer. The hormonal hyperstimulation as part of IVF also results in an endometrium, which is more hypertrophic than in unstimulated cycles in theory, rendering it less fit for trophoblast invasion, and this may increase the risk of early miscarriage. One study has shown that in IVF cycles with an endometrial thickness of >14 mm, the pregnancy rate is only 8% whereas the miscarriage rate was as high as 66% compared with 30% and 22%, respectively, in cycles with an endometrium thickness of 7–14 mm.

Excessive suppression of LH with GnRH agonists in the follicular phase of IVF cycles has also been suspected to increase the risk of subsequent miscarriage from 9% in cases with no/slight suppression to 45% in cases with strong suppression.

The in vitro culture of the embryos can in theory induce damage to the embryonal genome: the culture media may lack important nutrients or growth factors found in the tube and endometrium.

⚗ SCIENCE REVISITED

Recurrent miscarriages after ART may be due to the same factors causing the infertility problem – endocrine, endometriosis-related, male factor, tubal, or immunological abnormalities – but may also be caused by procedures related to IUI/IVF/ICSI treatment such as ovarian superovulation, endometrial hyperstimulation, excessive downregulation, or conditions relating to embryo culture.

Treatment

As is the case for almost all types of RM, there is no real documented treatment of RM associated with ART. Again we must consider the situation differently between patients treated with IUI or IVF/ICSI. In cases with recurrent PULs after IUI our first choice is to offer IVF because of the suspicion that the problem is due to recurrent spontaneously resorbed tubal pregnancies caused by subtotal tubal damage. More than half of the recurrent PUL patients in our clinic deliver after 1–2 IVF attempts, but clearly a randomized prospective study is needed to clarify the issue.

✋ CAUTION

A significant proportion of patients with recurrent pregnancy losses without histological or ultrasonic evidence of intrauterine pregnancy (PULs) may in fact suffer from recurrent tubal pregnancies rather than RMs and may benefit from IVF treatment solely.

In our clinic, several other options exist for treating RM patients with confirmed intrauterine pregnancy losses or RM after IVF/ICSI. One possibility is just to offer standard ART treatment without any modifications to these women. Alternatively, a more active approach is to provide (i) treatments that would be offered to RM patients with no conception problems and (ii) to modify ART treatment in order to diminish treatment-related factors that may be associated with an increased miscarriage rate. Our clinic favors the active approach.

The treatment options offered to patients with genuine RM after ART seek to normalize the presumed miscarriage-causing factors. In PCOS patients, we recommend weight loss to diminish obesity and offer treatment with estrogen-containing contraceptive pills before ART to suppress increased testosterone and LH levels. It seems logical to advise these patients to lose weight but there is still no proof from clinical trials that weight loss really decreases the future miscarriage rate. The same is true with regard to treatment with contraceptive pills before conception. Although it clearly normalizes plasma testosterone and LH levels in PCOS patients, still no prospective controlled trial has documented the effect of this therapy regarding the succeeding miscarriage rate.

In patients with endometriosis, treatments to reduce the peritoneal lesions – surgery and administration of estrogen-suppressing drugs – have been proven to increase the chance of conception but whether the miscarriage rate is diminished needs to be documented too.

In case of very poor sperm quality with and without detectable sperm chromatin abnormalities the use of IUI or IVF with a donor sperm could be considered, but again no studies have documented the effect on the miscarriage rate. Ongoing studies are investigating the possibility of isolating spermatozoa with normal sperm chromatin content for use in ICSI, but results from these are still awaited.

Large sacto-/hydrosalpinges visible by ultrasound in patients with no pregnancy or miscarriages after IVF/ICSI should be surgically removed, since there is documentation that this significantly improves the live birth rate from 16.3% in nonsurgically treated women to 28.6% in treated women. The increased live birth rate was primarily due to a 10% lower miscarriage rate in the latter group, suggesting that the presence of sacto-/hydrosalpinges created unfavorable uterine conditions for the embryos after implantation.

In case of poor ovarian reserve and advanced maternal age, the only treatment that probably both improves the implantation rate and diminishes the miscarriage rate is egg donation from a young donor.

As mentioned, there are many indications of a link between immunological disturbances and repeated implantation failure or miscarriages after ART; therefore special consideration should be given to various forms of immunotherapy.

Some prospective but not randomized studies have suggested that treatment with prednisone may increase the live birth rate by 15% in IVF patients with autoantibodies. However, a small but adequately randomized trial did not find that treatment with intravenous immunoglobulin (IvIg) improved the live birth rate in women with repeated implantation failure after IVF. In our clinic we offer combined treatment with 10 mg prednisone and IvIg starting before embryo transfer and continued till week 7 (prednisone) and week 14 (IvIg) in patients not selected due to any immunological abnormality (see Chapter 17). In 52 patients with RM after IVF/ICSI, this immunomodulation resulted in a live birth rate of 36.5% after the next IVF/ICSI treatment and

52.5% after three IVF/ICSI cycles combined with immunomodulation. Although these results must be tested in a placebo-controlled trial, the combination therapy proves promising in patients with RM after IVF/ICSI.

> **⚬ SCIENCE REVISITED**
>
> No treatment for RM after ART has been sufficiently documented except for oocyte donation in case of severe ovarian failure. However, treatment to improve endocrine conditions and immunotherapy can be empirically attempted but still lack real documentation. Changes of stimulation protocols or culture media may be attempted.

Concerning the causes of miscarriages assumed to be related to the ART technique, the procedures can be modified in order to diminish the putative risk factors.

Excessive superovulation should be avoided using low-stimulation protocols, and excessive LH suppression in the follicular phase can be avoided by using short GnRH antagonist protocols. A hyperstimulated endometrium could be avoided by freezing the embryos and transferring them into an unstimulated natural cycle. Finally, culture conditions for the embryos should reflect conditions in the in vivo situations as much as possible: culture media should be optimized to contain all important nutrients and growth factors of importance. A recent study has shown that addition of the growth factor/cytokine granulocyte-macrophage colony stimulating factor (GM-CSF) to IVF culture media seems to improve the ongoing pregnancy rate and diminish the miscarriage rate in patients with a history of miscarriage and infertility.

Bibliography

Harris, D.L. and Daniluk, J.C. (2010) The experience of spontaneous pregnancy loss for infertile women who have conceived through assisted reproduction technology. *Human Reproduction*, **25**, 714–720.

Hviid, T.V.F., Hylenius, S., Lindhard, A. and Christiansen, O.B. (2004) Association between human leukocyte antigen-G genotype and success of in-vitro fertilization and pregnancy outcome. *Tissue Antigens*, **64**, 66–69.

Robinson, L., Gallos, I.D., Conner, S.J. *et al* (2012) The effect of sperm DNA fragmentation on miscarriage rates: a systematic review and meta-analysis. *Human Reproduction*, **10**, 2908–2917.

Wang, J.X., Norman, R.J. and Wilcox, A.J. (2004) Incidence of spontaneous abortion among pregnancies produced by assisted reproductive technology. *Human Reproduction*, **19**, 272–277.

13

How to Cope with Stress and Depression in Women with Recurrent Miscarriage

Keren Shakhar and Dida Fleisig

Department of Behavioral Sciences, The College of Management Academic Studies, Rishon Le-Zion, Israel

Stress and depression in women with recurrent miscarriage

Recurrent miscarriage is much more than a Medical Condition

Becoming a mother is many women's desire from a very young age. After marriage, women often picture themselves having children and may have a clear idea of how many children they want, when they wish to have them, and at what intervals. They might also imagine how they or their partner would function as a parent. For them, pregnancy and labor are considered the most natural thing, and the idea that something may interfere with such plans rarely crosses their minds. Therefore, when a miscarriage occurs, many women and their spouses are shocked and feel that their major plans have been shuffled. When a second miscarriage occurs, they are often devastated, feel even more depressed, and fear that it might not be just bad luck. After a third miscarriage, many feel that their basic beliefs about themselves and their life have been shattered and that they are losing control over their bodies and their ability to plan their lives.

Since it is the women who physically experience the miscarriages, they are often most prone to emotional effects. Many women perceive their self-worth and identity to be depending on whether they succeed in having a child. Failing to stay pregnant makes these women feel defective, unwomanly, and betrayed by their own bodies. Additionally, the miscarriage itself may involve rapid hospitalization, massive bleeding and pain, and can potentially become a traumatic event. Hormonal changes after the miscarriage may also lead to emotional fluctuations as well as amplify existing emotions.

Although women are under the spotlight, recurrent miscarriage (RM) is usually a very painful and tolling experience for the male spouses as well. Because men are often less inclined than women to discuss their emotion, and because the medical examination is centered on the women, their pain often goes unnoticed. Men commonly try to cope by engaging themselves at work and trying to act rationally and be in control.

Recurrent Pregnancy Loss, First Edition. Edited by Ole B. Christiansen.
© 2014 John Wiley & Sons, Ltd. Published 2014 by John Wiley & Sons, Ltd.

RM may occur at different stages in a couple's relationship and may raise different emotions. If it occurs before they have had a child, it may lead to fear of never having a biological child. When secondary miscarriages occur, couples may perceive it as hurting the existing child's well-being. They feel responsible for failing to provide the child with a sibling and may feel guilty that their child is alone and the age gap with the desired child is increasing. Thus, although the way RM affects the couple depends on whether it is primary or secondary, the experience is overwhelming and upsetting for all.

> **PATIENT ADVICE**
>
> Help the couple understand that many women with RM occasionally experience intensive emotional turbulences and that this is a common part of the grieving process.
>
> Many women are unaware that their emotional reaction is a common response to RMs and fear that they are losing their sanity.

Anxiety and Depression are Common Responses to RM

Approximately a third of all couples with RM experience severe depression and many more experience anxiety at least once during the course. Such depression and anxiety can last several months and even a year and may be accompanied by symptoms such as frequent weeping with apparently no external or internal reason, lethargy, having no motivation to carry daily tasks, sleeping too much or too little, increased or reduced appetite, and diminished interest in social events. Even when women are not depressed they may experience sudden fluctuations in emotions. A typical response of women to RM is feeling fine and in control one moment and bursting into tears the next. Often there is a trigger for their emotions which they are not aware of (e.g., a commercial about babies on TV, seeing a child cross the street, or arrival of a due date that is not relevant anymore). Since many women do not expect their emotions to be so strong and do not consider their reaction normal, they feel overwhelmed and sometimes even fear for their psychological health.

During pregnancy, women with RM may become extremely anxious as they feel little confidence in their ongoing pregnancy and in their body. In contrast to women with a single miscarriage, the fear of losing the baby does not decline to control level after the first trimester or when they pass the week of gestation in prior miscarriages. Women may be repeatedly looking for signs that the embryo is still alive and may find themselves obsessively checking for bleeding, getting upset by any abdominal pain, and worrying if any of the first trimester physical signs (e.g., nausea, fatigue, etc.) disappears. Intrusive thoughts about pregnancy are common and may be most intense during the night when they are less busy. In order to minimize such fears and worries women often try to avoid fantasies about the embryo and consequently feel less attached to it. Magical thinking and superstitious rituals may also be common.

How anxious and depressed couples feel largely depends on how they interpret the events and frame for themselves what had happened to them. Although miscarriage itself is an objective event, different meaning and weight could be ascribed to it, leading to different emotions. Several studies have shown that women who invest in other domains of life such as personal goals, women who place greater value on their relationship with their spouse, and women who attribute less significance to the miscarriage are more immune to the emotional upsetting effects of RM. In addition, moderate age, positive self-esteem, and higher sociodemographic status are also related to better adjustment to infertility.

The Grieving Process

Although not recognized as so, when couples grieve over their lost embryo, it is in many ways similar to the grief experienced over the loss of a close relative. They have often already viewed their embryo as a baby, nicknamed him, and felt love toward him. The loss is encompassing many aspects of life. Besides the loss of a child, of being called mom and dad, couples often lose their transition to parenthood, they lose a dream, and they lose the fun they had with their family friends and the joyful experience of pregnancies. Women also often lose their feeling of womanhood, their ability to plan and trust their bodies, their identity, and self-confidence.

⚜ SCIENCE REVISITED

Although many lay people are not aware, miscarriage is a tragic event for most women who experience it. In the past years it has been increasingly recognized that most women (and their spouses) mourn the loss and that their response is similar in many aspects to that of a loss of a close family member.

Although this loss is encircling many facets of life, its grief differs in several ways from the grief over a dead child. As mentioned earlier, this grief is often private and regards someone the couples have never really met. Moreover, there is little acknowledgment from society to this loss and couples may find themselves expected to quickly adjust back to normal life. There is often no recognition that they may need some days off work, and there are no rituals such as burial or a ceremony to structure the mourning or provide the grieving couple with social support. Last, unlike other grieving processes, this grief is accompanied by women's hormonal changes that by themselves can lead to emotional instability.

This gap between couples' emotional response to the loss and the obliviousness demonstrated by society may at times raise fears concerning the normality of their emotional response. Couples may be unaware that they are grieving and may be bewildered by the strength and length of their emotions. Although studies show that men usually grieve for a shorter period, it is unclear what the normal trajectory of grieving in RM is. It is likely that most couples will probably go through the five stages which were described by Kubler Ross. These stages have been accepted and generalized to a wide variety of losses. Here is a short description of how these stages can surface in couples with RM:

1. Shock/denial – This is usually the first response to the loss and is characterized by numbness and disbelief that this is really happening. Couples may seem as if they are ignorant to the loss.

2. Anger – Many couples feel that life is unfair and question why the miscarriages happened to them of all people. They may be angry and feel that they stir up inside. This anger could be pointed to anyone including family, friends, themselves, or the physician.
3. Yearning – Yearning or deep longing to the embryo may be the most salient symptom of grief.
4. Depression – Couples may feel very sad and lonely and may find themselves crying frequently. Also, it may be difficult for them to concentrate and they may feel very fatigued to do any daily task.
5. Acceptance – Couples at this stage face reality and try to attribute a different meaning to what happened to them, so they can move on with their life. Clues that the couple has reached this point include realizing that they are not the only ones experiencing RM, and being a little encouraged that since others made it through, so can they.

RM is a very Lonely Experience

When people endure a crisis in life, social support can help them cope with the situation as well as buffer the effects of stress. Unfortunately for many couples suffering from RM, the experience is accompanied by collapse in support systems. Their friends and family may not even be aware that they are experiencing miscarriages. Often, there is a lot of secrecy around pregnancy especially during the first trimester, and couples may experience the miscarriages before they had shared their pregnancy with their friends and family. In addition, many women feel ashamed and embarrassed to talk about their miscarriages. They fear they will not be understood and are unsure how to communicate the situation and their emotions. Even when the experience is shared with others, women may feel that their loss is played down and not recognized. Such emotions often mount when friends respond with recommendations of what to do and what not to do, or with statements such as "at least you know you can get pregnant" or "maybe it's good that this baby was lost, it was probably defected." Although their friends mean good when making such statements, they often make couples with RM feel that they are judged and criticized, in addition to not receiving any emotional support.

As more miscarriages occur and the couples' need for support intensifies, their social relationships with friends often dwindle. Insensitive remarks are only one reason for the disruption in relationships. Additional causes relate to the fact that their friends are entering a stage in life in which babies and children become central topics of discussion. Such topics are not only strange to couples with RM, but are also painful reminders of their losses. While engaged in these conversations, couples with RM may find themselves pretending that everything is OK while deep inside they feel that life is falling apart. Since discussing such matters becomes unbearable, couples may refrain from going to events or places where they might run into children, pregnant women, or discussion about such subjects. Eventually, at a time when social support is most needed, couples may feel isolated from their family and close friends.

In addition to the loss of their support systems, couples and especially women may be surprised by new emotions that emerge toward their friends. Anger, bitterness, and jealousy are very common among women. Questions regarding fairness in life may cross their minds. Couples are often not aware that those are normal responses to their circumstances and may feel guilty and ashamed for having such socially unaccepted emotions and thoughts. Many couples try to hide these feelings and may be very frustrated with their experience.

Since couples sometimes cannot rely on previous support systems, they struggle to find new ones. They tend to assume that that they can be understood only by those who have had a similar experience. Yet, finding such couples is not easy. First, not many couples talk about it. Second, it is often hard to get acquainted with other women sharing the same problem at the clinic as there is often no separate unit for women with RM. Last, there are very few support groups in the internet that are unique to RM.

Internet forums and blogs can serve as a good source of emotional support. Women use them much more frequently than men, and they report using these forums mainly to get empathy, warmth, understanding, sense of belonging, and to share their feelings. When a study evaluated themes in internet forums for pregnancy loss, the theme that was by far the most common was "I'm not alone in the experience." Women use these sites to assure themselves that they are not alone. It is a stage where women can meet other women experiencing a similar situation as well as find reassurance that their strong emotions are normal, that their thoughts are typical and not bad, and that others still accept them and do not resent them despite those thoughts and feelings. Not all women who visit forums and blogs are active visitors. Many of them are just silent readers but, nonetheless, it can still grant them some of the emotional support they desperately need.

PATIENT ADVICE

Provide couples with internet forum sites that specifically address RM. Although these forums are relatively scarce, here are few examples for active forums in the English language:

http://forums.fertilitycommunity.com/recurrent-miscarriages/

http://community.babycentre.co.uk/groups/a164715/recurrent_miscarriage_support

http://forums.ivillage.com/t5/Recurrent-Pregnancy-Loss/ct-p/iv-bhpregloss

Marital Relationship

RM has the potential to both strengthen marital relationship as well as increase tension and conflicts. Couples may feel united in their desire to have kids, in their grief, and in their difficulties coping. But at times they may also find it difficult to communicate their emotions, needs, desires, and fears. They may divert in their motivation to have kids and in the way they cope with the situation. While women may tend to repeatedly discuss the situation and express their emotions, men tend to be more action oriented and bury themselves at work.

★ TIPS AND TRICKS

Try to involve the male partner in the treatment: put his name on the file, address him during the appointment and encourage him to come.

Many women with RM feel that they cope alone. Such an approach can involve the partner more, and help women feel less lonely.

Such divergence in coping styles may lead to many misunderstandings. Women may interpret their partner's response as uncaring and unloving. As a result they may start looking for signs of affection (e.g., calls, hugs, etc.) that will reassure them that he still loves them. They may feel responsible for the rupture in relationship and may relate it to their inability to carry pregnancy to terms or to their strong emotional response to it. Men on the other hand may perceive their role as protecting and may seek ways to comfort their wives and hide their own emotions. They are often worried about their wives' psychological well-being and try to comfort them by saying the "right" words, and pretending to be strong by hiding their true feelings. They are often not aware that what many women need is to share their pain and to know that the RMs influence their spouses' emotions as well.

Decision making and its relation to stress and depression

Couples experiencing RM face the need to make a variety of decisions during their usually extended difficult situation: having to decide whether to continue with their physician or go to a specialist; wishing to choose or at least to participate in the choice of treating the miscarriage; choosing or considering optional forthcoming treatments; and (eventually) having to decide when or whether to continue trying for further pregnancies.

Almost any decision making process bears potential feelings of discomfort and at times even stress, anxiety, and a feeling of loss of control over one's life. These feelings are intensified by the perceived importance of the decision and by the ambiguity or insufficiency of the information upon which the decision is made. Moreover, decision making often involves risk – that is, potentially choosing an action that could lead to undesirable results – which increases stress and anxiety. Feelings of stress affect not only the decision makers' well-being but also the decision's quality, as informed decisions require unbiased thinking based on the most comprehensive and relevant information available.

Decision processes experienced by couples with RM start – as decision processes usually do – with the need to identify the problem, that is, to recognize the causes of the miscarriage. Even if couples are not really interested in the causes per se, they keep searching for them in hope of increasing the chances of a successful future pregnancy. Consequently couples with RM are ready to undergo almost any examination that may indicate what their problem is. When causes are not fully or indisputably recognized, couples experience an increase in levels of stress, hopelessness, and depression.

The following step in the decision process calls for gathering information concerning treatment alternatives and optional actions, including risks and side effects. Choices are made according to the decision makers' preferences and goals, yet as couples frequently hold many and occasionally conflicting preferences, stress or anxiety might rise. The couples' foremost goal is having a biological child, however, health issues, psychological states, moral, ethical, and social concerns very often pose conflicting goals and hinder establishing clear preferences, thus adding to feelings of distress and uncertainty.

People often base their probabilistic evaluations of a future event on the ease with which relevant instances come to their minds, eventually leading to biased judgments (the Availability Heuristic, Tversky and Kahneman, 1973).

When considering risky choices, people often apply biased reasoning, as when granting disproportional high probabilities to events which occurred more recently, were more salient, vivid, or emotionally laden; or when focusing on outcomes and ways to control or avoid them, while ignoring the probabilities of their occurrences. Moreover, the way risky choices are presented – the framing of information – has a massive effect on the choice itself. Physicians can present potential outcomes as the percentage of a treatment's success or as the probability of its failure. For instance, positive framing that emphasized the absence of disease (e.g., saying that among 100 women, breast cancer will not develop in 95 of them in the next 15 years) might evoke less willingness to participate in treatment than negative framing (e.g., among 100 women, breast cancer will develop in 5 women in the next 15 years). Understanding numerical expression of risk and probability are quite difficult, as most people interpret words better than numbers. For example, risk conveyed in the form of percentage (e.g., your risk of receiving a diagnosis of breast cancer within the next 5 years is 1.1%) is usually less understood than when formulated in a more descriptive form (e.g., among 1000 women with similar characteristics, 11 would receive a diagnosis of breast cancer within the next 5 years, whereas 989 would not). However, the preference for literal rather than numerical expressions might lead to a biased perception of probabilities, such as when reducing probabilities into binary categories of "low risk" and "high risk," (e.g., "the chance of keeping the pregnancy is 10 % vs. the chance of keeping the pregnancy is low"), thus enabling patients a big variety of interpretation, distorting the perception of risk and hence the decision itself.

✋ CAUTION

Beware of Framing Effects

Decision makers might shift their preference because of the way choices are framed.

Shared decision making is a contemporary patient-centered decision making approach in which patients and clinicians actively and mutually consider options, preferences, and probabilities, resulting in a consensual healthcare decision. The clinicians' duty is to provide accurate and relevant information, as patients frequently introduce and base their decisions on information randomly gathered from medical internet-sights, forums, and blogs. Such information is frequently unreliable as it is often anecdotal, or based on attention-capturing extreme cases that raise emotions and are better remembered – yet should not be generalized or based upon. The shared decision making process also aims to encourage patients to take an active role in managing their health. Indeed, patients who were involved in shared decision processes were more satisfied, more adherent to treatment, and reported higher well-being and greater perception of control over their lives, compared to patients participating in traditional clinical decision processes.

How can clinicians assist in decision processes and improve coping?

As already stated, RM is much more than a medical condition, bearing feelings of distress, loneliness, anxiety, and depression. Its effects are often long lasting, requiring many choices and decisions along the way, often intensifying distress because of uncertainty and lack of knowledge. We, hereafter, suggest possible coping support strategies to assist in decision making processes and present tips that can help alleviate psychological stress and depression.

How can Clinicians Assist in Decision Processes?

Responsible and cautious joint decisions can be achieved by providing the relevant information and by letting the patients raise any questions and express any concerns they have. Clinicians are advised to communicate risk very cautiously. It can be achieved by turning raw risky data into more understandable information such as by using visual aids like pie charts. Because of framing effects, clinicians are recommended to present patients with both – positive and negative – frames ("65 out of 100 chance of success" and "35 out of 100 chance of failure") in order to enable an unbiased perception of risky choices.

> **PATIENT ADVICE**
>
> As patients should be presented with full yet unbiased information, communicate risky outcomes very cautiously by presenting probabilities with visual aids, and by framing outcomes positively as well as negatively.

Couples dealing with infertility problems bring into their decision considerations a variety of values, thus physicians are advised to recognize all those values, and allow them to be incorporated into the decision making processes.

One of the most difficult decisions couples with RM have to make is whether to stop trying to have their biological child, as it eventually leads to giving up that dream. This difficult decision is in most cases complicated by conflicting emotions and information, and by pressure from family and society. It is important to keep in mind that even when physicians' advice is asked for, the final decision, whether to proceed trying to have a natural pregnancy or to consider various other options, is the couples' decision and not the physicians' choice.

How can Clinicians Improve Coping with Stress and Depression?

Many clinicians recognize the emotional burden RM puts on couples; however, they are unsure how they can psychologically assist the couples in the very limited time they have. Although couples usually do not expect their clinicians to have psychological tools to assist them to cope with the situation, they often report that they do wish their clinicians would listen and respect them, that they will feel that their clinician cares about them and desperately desires that they will have a baby.

Here are a few brief tips that can be used in the clinic to improve not only the couples' well-being but also the clinician's rapport with them:

1. Since there is often no certain cause for the miscarriage, some women believe they did something that might have caused the miscarriage. Make sure they do not blame themselves for what had happened. This can be done by checking with them the causes they believe underlie their miscarriages.

2. Be emphatic to their pain and inform them that depression and anxiety are normal and typical reactions to their losses. Part of the couples' depression and anxiety often results from their fear that their responses are extreme and do not emanate directly from the losses themselves. Such reassurance can comfort them that they are normal as well as make them feel that they are understood and that the impact the miscarriages have on them is acknowledged.

3. Some couples fear getting pregnant again because of the threat of re-experiencing the negative emotional responses in case of an additional miscarriage. That fear might overshadow all other considerations concerning future pregnancies. Assure couples that their fear is legitimate and normal in those circumstances and advise them to get counseling to better deal with their anxiety.

4. As anxiety levels climb up during pregnancy, women may feel it is necessary to inform their clinician and discuss issues related to pregnancy such as treatment, monitoring, and precautions about lifestyles and diet during pregnancy. Many women prefer to be treated, especially at this crucial time, by one physician. If possible, encourage such an appointment with you once they are pregnant. If not, make sure they know when to schedule the first appointment and why it is not necessary to do so earlier.

5. If possible offer women repeated ultrasounds every week or two while pregnant. Some women want to assure themselves that their fetus is still alive. Yet, it is important to remember that the time before ultrasounds checks is very stressful and women may be very nervous.

6. Try to involve the male partner. This can be done by directly addressing him, placing his name on the file as well and encouraging him to attend all medical appointments.

What Types of Emotional Supports can Infertility Centers Provide to Women with RM?

Apart from the support received in the physician's office, there are additional steps that centers for RM can take to help couples adjust better to the adverse experience of RM. These include providing support throughout the abortion process itself, as well as offering counseling services and various psychological tools that can enhance later coping.

When a miscarriage occurs it sometimes involves hospitalization and curettage. At some centers dilation and curettage are often not scheduled to the next day and women may find themselves walking with a dead embryo for several days. Many women find that idea hard to tolerate. If curettage cannot be scheduled early, its psychological deleterious effects should at least be recognized.

While hospitalized, women are sometimes placed in the same unit and even room as women who are considered at high risk. This is a very difficult situation for both sides. Women who have just lost their dream may find it hard to discuss their pain with pregnant women and find it very difficult to be empathic to them. For women at high risk, women with a miscarriage reflect their scariest dream. Avoiding such situations can ease the pain for both sides.

Although dilation and curettage are considered safe and simple medical procedures, they can be very stressful and perceived as humiliating for women experiencing them. Since women are often under general anesthesia, they are not aware of what is done during the procedure and often report feelings of loss of control. Meeting with the surgeon and the medical team to discuss these matters prior to the procedure can lower anxiety levels for some women. A constant figure that will meet the couple throughout the whole procedure can also comfort the couple and make them feel more familiar with the team.

After the procedure ends, couples are sent home to recover. As in many other medical procedures, couples may experience side effects and emotional turbulences and feel that they have no one to turn to. Providing them with personal contact information is essential and is something couples express desire for. Discussing possible causes for the miscarriage, its potential implications, and letting them discuss their emotions at this follow up is essential and can significantly lower their anxiety levels. Most women prefer this meeting to be with a clinician.

In addition to following the whole process of miscarriage, it is advisable for the center to offer couples various techniques to alleviate the negative effects of stress. If such programs cannot be provided within a center it is recommended to refer the couples to such support. Here are a few examples of support that can be given at a center.

Relaxation Training

The relaxation response is a physical state in which bodily and emotional responses to stress are reduced. It is characterized by slower breathing, lower blood pressure and heart rate, and more peaceful mood. Such relaxed responses can be brought about by various techniques that can be quickly and easily learned in a group setting or individually. These techniques include guided imagery or focusing on breathing or phrases, body scan, or progressive muscle relaxation. Relaxation techniques have been shown to control hypertension and headaches. After learning the techniques, couples can elicit the relaxation response by themselves or by tape whenever they feel the need.

Cognitive Behavioral Therapy

The idea behind cognitive behavioral therapy is that what we think affects how we feel. Many of our cognitive responses to stressful situations are automatic and involve irrational thoughts. Such erroneous thoughts can increase stress and lead to depression and anxiety. In cognitive behavioral therapy patients learn to recognize such irrational thoughts, to challenge their rationality, and finally to restructure them into more truthful and positive thoughts, leading eventually to improved emotional states.

For example, in response to a miscarriage a woman might think "I'll never be a mom." Challenging such thoughts involves checking the truth of this statement. A more positive and truthful statement will be "I might experience another miscarriage but there is also a good chance that I will eventually succeed in having babies."

Support Groups

Support groups bring together couples with similar experiences and therefore can provide the couples with a sense that their feeling and concerns are shared and understood. As many couples with RM experience loneliness and seclusion, support groups can ease those feelings and assure couples that their emotional responses and thoughts are common and normal.

Conclusions

RM is one of the most devastating fertility problems and is characterized by repeated episodes of anxiety, depression, and complex decision making processes. Probably, more than in any other fertility problem, the couples' pain is not properly acknowledged by society and they feel secluded and lonely. At present, proper and available places to receive the needed emotional support are scarce. However there are various ways in which fertility centers can assist such couples alleviate the pain they experience, help them cope, and facilitate their decisions processes. Such interventions can be briefly given by the physician during a medical appointment or more comprehensively by various caregivers in the fertility center.

Bibliography

Geller, P.A., Psaros, C. and Kornfield, S.L. (2010) Satisfaction with pregnancy loss aftercare: are women getting what they want? *Archives of Women's Mental Health*, **13** (2), 111–124.

Greil, A.L., Slauson-Blevins, K. and McQuillan, J. (2010) The experience of infertility: a review of recent literature. *Sociology of Health & Illness*, **32** (1), 140–162.

Tversky, A. and Kahneman, D. (1981) The framing of decisions and the psychology of choice. *Science (New York)*, **211** (4481), 453–458.

14

Recurrent Miscarriage and the Risk of Autoimmune Disease and Thromboembolic Disease

M. Angeles Martínez-Zamora,[1] Ricard Cervera[2] and Juan Balasch[1]

[1] Institute Clínic of Gynecology, Obstetrics and Neonatology, Hospital Clínic, University of Barcelona, Barcelona, Catalonia, Spain
[2] Department of Autoimmune Diseases, Institute Clínic of Medicine and Dermatology, Hospital Clínic, University of Barcelona, Barcelona, Catalonia, Spain

Introduction

The relationship between recurrent miscarriage (RM) and both autoimmunity and hemostatic abnormalities has long been recognized. On one side, because most autoimmune disturbances have a predilection for women in their reproductive years, the clinical impact of abnormal autoimmune function on reproductive processes has a paramount importance. More specifically, several studies have reported the presence of various autoantibodies (i.e., antithyroid and antiphospholipid antibodies (aPL)) in patients with unexplained RM and some autoimmune diseases (i.e., systemic lupus erythematosus (SLE) and the antiphospholipid syndrome (APS)) present a higher prevalence of RM than the general population. However, the questions arise as to which autoantibodies should be sought in women with unexplained RM, and which antibodies are clearly predictive of RM in patients with known autoimmune diseases.

On the other hand, the hemostatic pathways are intimately involved in ovulation, implantation, and placentation. Pregnancy itself has long been recognized as being a hypercoagulable state, characterized by an increase in the levels of certain coagulation factors, a decrease in the levels of anticoagulant proteins, and an increase in fibrinolysis. The evolutionary advantage of this hypercoagulability may be to counteract the inherent instability associated with hemochorial placentation, which is unique to human beings. However, it is well known that many cases of miscarriage, both early and late, are caused by an exaggerated hemostatic response during pregnancy, leading to thrombosis of the placental vasculature and subsequent pregnancy loss. Recent insight into RM pathogenesis has proposed a different view of thrombotic events in RM patients. It has been hypothesized that occult cardiovascular, microvascular, or hemostatic dysfunction results in pregnancy complications during reproductive

Recurrent Pregnancy Loss, First Edition. Edited by Ole B. Christiansen.
© 2014 John Wiley & Sons, Ltd. Published 2014 by John Wiley & Sons, Ltd.

years and in thrombotic disease later in life. Therefore, a woman's reproductive history may inform on future thrombosis risk. The aforementioned notwithstanding, a key question arises: Do RM patients have a higher risk of thrombosis later in life?

In this chapter, we will analyze all these challenging questions regarding RM and the risk of autoimmune or thromboembolic disease.

RM and autoimmunity

Although a number of autoantibodies have been occasionally linked to RM, only the aPL have been clearly associated to RM both in patients with a known autoimmune disease – that is, the APS or SLE – and in the general population. In the latter, about 10% of patients with RM are found to have aPL. This is a substantial percentage, considering that genetic and anatomical factors, the well-accepted causes of RM, are together detected in only 5–15% of patients.

RM and aPL

The APS – a condition that combines arterial and venous thrombosis, obstetric morbidity, and the presence of aPL and which can be primary or associated to SLE – is the autoimmune disease most commonly associated with RM. Furthermore, a large number of studies have found that in women with SLE, those with aPL are at increased risk for RM. However, the incidence of RM in the APS and in SLE has been reported as varying from as high as 90% to as low as 15%.

⚙ SCIENCE REVISITED

The APS – a condition that combines arterial and venous thrombosis, obstetric morbidity and the presence of aPL and which can be primary or associated to SLE – is the autoimmune disease most commonly associated with RM. Furthermore, a large number of studies have found that in women with SLE, those with aPL are at increased risk for RM. However, the incidence of RM in the APS and in SLE has been reported as varying from as high as 90% to as low as 15%.

Controversy still remains over the type (early or late) of pregnancy loss more closely related with aPL. However, both clinical and experimental data using APS animal models support the evidence that any type of pregnancy loss (including preimplantation embryos), but mainly embryo resorption, may be associated with aPL.

The association of aPL and RM in patients with SLE and the APS suggests a causative role but, by no means, it does prove it. The major pregnancy-related target for aPL is the placenta and utero-placental insufficiency is often attributed to vasculopathy of the terminal spiral arteries which nourish the placentary intervillous space. These vessels had smaller diameter and showed intimal layer thickening, fibrinoid necrosis, and intraluminal thrombosis. In other cases, the infarcted region may show villous congestion and hemorrhage and early trophoblastic necrosis. In addition to placental infarction and thrombosis, perivillous fibrin deposition and evidence of decidua vascular atherosis, indicative of spiral artery vasculopathy, are seen in some

APS cases. All these findings are, however, not specific to APS and do not always correlate with the fetal outcome.

The mechanisms by which aPL may cause the earlier-described changes are not completely understood and several hypotheses have been proposed. For instance, aPL may interfere with the function of natural inhibitors of coagulation such as placental anticoagulant proteins (PAP) and others. PAP are a group of four calcium-dependent phospholipid-binding proteins that inhibit phospholipid-dependent steps of coagulation by making phospholipid inaccessible to clotting factors. The major component of the PAP family is the PAP-1, also called annexin V, which is most abundant in the placenta. Annexin V and aPL compete for phospholipids in coagulation assays. It has been shown that distribution of annexin V over the intervillous surface was significantly lower in patients with APS than in women with RM due to other causes. These findings suggest that reduced annexin V production and inhibition of its anticoagulant function by aPL may play a role in pregnancy loss in APS patients.

However, other nonthrombotic mechanisms have been implicated, interference with the embryonic implantation being the one that has received more attention. The aPL have been found to react directly with third trimester villous trophoblast cells, prevent proliferation of trophoblast derived from choriocarcinoma cells, inhibit in vitro chemotaxis and differentiation of villous trophoblast isolated from third trimester placentae, decrease trophoblast invasion, and inhibit extravillous trophoblast differentiation. Furthermore, aPL can induce pregnancy loss in mice by impairing the embryonic implantation capacity, likely because a direct interaction with the trophectoderm cells.

Additionally, aPL may impair the placentary production of chorionic gonadotropin during the early phases of pregnancy, thus determining the embryonic evolution and, in the mice model, APS is associated with a diminished secretion of interleukin-3, positively related with pregnancy, and the pregnancy loss is prevented by in vitro administration of recombinant interleukin-3.

Recently, the role of complement activation by the aPL has also received a great deal of attention. Several studies have suggested that activation of the complement cascade is necessary for aPL-mediated thrombophilia and RM. In mice, it was found that inhibition of the complement cascade *in vivo*, using the C3 convertase inhibitor complement receptor 1-related gene protein y (Crry)-Ig, blocks aPL-induced fetal loss and growth retardation and reversed aPL-mediated thrombosis. Furthermore, mice deficient in complement C3 and C5 (C3–/– and C5–/–, respectively) were resistant to thrombosis, endothelial cell activation and fetal loss induced by aPL. Additionally, an anti-C5 monoclonal antibody reversed thrombogenic properties of aPL in vivo, then confirming the involvement of C5 complement activation in aPL-induced thrombosis. It has also been shown that the interaction of complement component 5a (C5a) with its receptor (C5aR) is necessary for thrombosis of placental vasculature.

RM and other autoantibodies

In addition to aPL, several other autoantibodies have been occasionally related to unexplained RM, including antithyroid, antiannexin V, antiprothrombin, antinuclear, antilaminin, and IgA and IgG antigliadin and IgA antitransglutaminase antibodies related to celiac disease.

In a study of 38 women with unexplained RM and 28 control parous women, the authors found a significant association between unexplained RM and antithyroid peroxidase antibodies and a combinational panel of autoantibodies, including those against thyroid peroxidase, thyroglobulin, and extractable nuclear antigens, but not with aPL. However, the data on the association of antithyroid antibodies and RM are conflicting and a statistically significant association has not been shown in other large studies. In another study, our group analyzed 109 patients with RM and 120 healthy women. In RM, aPL, antiprothrombin, and anti-*Saccharomyces cerevisiae* antibodies were more prevalent than in controls, with an odds ratio (OR) of 4.8, 5.4, and 3.9 for each antibody, respectively.

Therefore, although there is a general consensus to screen for aPL in patients with RM, larger cohort studies are necessary to determine the true incidence of RM in the presence of other autoantibody or combinations of autoantibodies. Cohorts of healthy women with no previous obstetric problems should be screened for autoantibodies and followed prospectively to register whether those with autoantibodies miscarry their future pregnancies more often than those without. In addition, these cohort studies should either be corrected for the subsequent miscarriages caused by fetal chromosomal aberrations, or use multivariate analysis to correct for the effect of confounding factors such as maternal age.

★ TIPS AND TRICKS

There is a general consensus to screen for aPL in patients with RM.

However, larger cohort studies are necessary to determine the true incidence of RM in the presence of other autoantibody or combinations of autoantibodies, and their routine determination cannot be recommended.

RM, aPL, and the Risk of Autoimmune Disease

So far, no prospective studies have adequately studied the risk of development of a full-blown autoimmune disease after RM, except in the case of RM associated to the presence of aPL. This topic was addressed by the "Euro-Phospholipid" project, a multicenter prospective study of 1000 patients with APS that were followed up during 5 years. Three out of 121 (2.5%) women with only RM (no history of previous thrombosis) and aPL (lupus anticoagulant and/or anticardiolipin antibodies) at the beginning of the study developed a new thrombotic event during the 5-year study period but none of them developed a full-blown SLE. Therefore, although the information is unfortunately scarce, it seems that the risk of development of SLE should be very low, but there is a risk of development of full-blown APS with thrombotic events and this will be discussed in the next section.

⚛ SCIENCE REVISITED

The risk of development of SLE after RM is apparently very low, but there is a certain risk of development of full-blown APS with thrombotic events.

RM and thromboembolic disease

Hemostatic Changes in RM Patients

Few prospective longitudinal studies have been published documenting changes in hemostatic variables in pregnant women with a history of RM. However, some studies provide evidence of abnormalities in the hemostatic pathways preceding fetal loss. It has been reported that women with a history of RM at 4–7 weeks of gestation have an excess of thromboxane production, and between weeks 8 and 11 they are relatively prostacyclin deficient, compared with women with no previous history of pregnancy loss. These changes were greatest among those whose pregnancy ended in miscarriage. The shift in the thromboxane to prostacyclin ratio in favor of the pro-thrombotic agent thromboxane may lead to vasospasm and platelet aggregation in the trophoblast, causing the development of microthrombi and placental necrosis.

Other studies also reported that changes in the hemostatic system preceded spontaneous abortion. For instance, the cases of two women have been reported in whom a significant decrease in the level of protein C and shortening in the rate of fibrinopeptide A generation (indicating activation of coagulation) could be detected several weeks in advance of miscarriage. In the second pregnancy of one of these two women, similar hematological changes were documented. These were reversed by the administration of heparin. The patient went on to deliver at term. Moreover, in a longitudinal study of pregnant women with APS, pregnancy in patients with significantly higher levels of thrombin–antithrombin complexes, a global marker of thrombotic potential, ended more frequently in miscarriage compared with those with an uncomplicated pregnancy.

Are Nonpregnant Women with a History of RM in a Prothrombotic State?

In a study by our group, Martínez-Zamora *et al.* (2012) reported that, outside of pregnancy, a group of women with first trimester RM are in a prothrombotic state, manifested by an impaired fibrinolytic response. It has also been reported, using global markers of the hemostatic process, that women with RM have increased thrombin generation and an increased maximum clot strength before pregnancy. Furthermore, women in such a state are at significantly increased risk of miscarriage in future untreated pregnancies.

⚜ SCIENCE REVISITED

A subgroup of women with RM has been demonstrated to be in a prothrombotic state before pregnancy. Furthermore, women in such a state are at significantly increased risk of miscarriage in future untreated pregnancies. The long-term health implications of this hypercoagulability have been highlighted in a large retrospective study reporting an increased risk of ischemic heart disease among women with a history of pregnancy loss.

The long-term health consequences of this hypercoagulability are being increasingly recognized; thus, it may imply an increased risk of ischemic heart disease in the subgroup of women with a history of RM. In a retrospective study of 130 000 women, Smith *et al.* (2001) reported that a history of first trimester spontaneous miscarriage was associated with a significant increased risk of maternal ischemic heart disease. This risk increased with the number of miscarriages such that among those with three or more miscarriages the risk of death or hospital admission for ischemic heart disease was 2.3 times greater than that among those with no previous history of miscarriage. In contrast, there was no association between therapeutic abortion and the subsequent risk of ischemic heart disease. The authors hypothesized that this may reflect common determinants, such as thrombophilic genetic defects or the presence of aPL. Clearly, if these retrospective data are confirmed in a large prospective study, pregnancy history will become an important criterion in the risk assessment of ischemic heart disease. Moreover, these findings may explain the results of previous studies that found an association between the total number of pregnancies (including births, miscarriages, and fetal deaths) and maternal risk of ischemic heart disease, as women who suffer RM must have more pregnancies to achieve their target family size.

In contrast, in a case-control study evaluating the long-term risk for thromboembolic events after RM, Martínez-Zamora *et al.* (2012) did not find a higher risk of thromboembolic events among idiopathic RM patients (idiopathic RM patients tested negative for genetic thrombophilias or aPL). This subject is further discussed later in the section "RM, aPL, and risk of thrombotic events."

The long-term risk of thrombotic events after pregnancy among patients with RM associated with inherited thrombophilic factors has been rarely evaluated. A previous study analyzing the long-term risk of RM patients concluded that the incidence of thrombosis was similar in the APS-negative RM group and in the APS-positive RM group (incidence of thrombosis: 2/1000 women-years vs. 6/1000 women-years, respectively). Both patients who developed a thrombotic event in the group without APS in the aforementioned study were found to be heterozygous for the Leiden factor V mutation or homozygous for the prothrombin gene mutation 20210A. This suggests that inherited thrombophilia factors may be risk factors for subsequent thrombotic events in RM patients. Moreover, recently, in another work by our group, Martínez-Zamora *et al.* (2012) performed a case-control study evaluating the long-term risk for thromboembolic events after RM in APS patients (cases: RM associated with the presence of aPL; controls: (i) idiopathic RM patients, (ii) RM patients with thrombophilic genetic disorders, and (iii) healthy aPL positive women without obstetric or thrombotic complications), and we found a higher risk, although not statistically significant, of thromboembolic events in the control group comprising RM patients who tested positive only for genetic thrombophilias compared with the idiopathic RM patients. The control group of RM patients with thrombophilic genetic defects as the only etiologic factor for their pregnancy losses consisted of 42 patients with three or more consecutive spontaneous abortions before 10 weeks gestation. Thrombophilia in this group was defined as factor V Leiden mutation in 17 patients, prothrombin G20210A gene mutation in 12 patients, protein C deficiency in 9 patients, or protein S deficiency in 4 patients. No woman in this group had combined thrombophilia (two or more findings), and thus, all tested negative for aPL. The idiopathic RM control group was composed of 86 patients with three or more consecutive spontaneous abortions who tested negative after routine screening for systemic diseases, diabetes mellitus, thyroid dysfunction, polycystic ovary disease, a chromosome assessment of the woman and her partner, uterine abnormalities, endometrial and hormonal luteal phase defects, endometrial and cervical infection, and thrombophilia (plasma levels of protein S and C, antithrombin, factor V Leiden, prothrombin G202010A mutation, acquired protein C resistance, and aPL). No patients in the idiopathic RM group (0%) and two patients in the thrombophilic genetic defects group (4.8%) presented with thrombotic events in the 12-year follow-up. The thrombophilic genetic defects group had 7.1 thrombotic events per 1000 patient-years, which is within the range of estimated risk reported in the literature for patients with inherited thrombophilia. This matter is further discussed in the next section.

RM, aPL, and Risk of Thrombotic Events

In contrast to venous thromboses associated with congenital thrombophilias, thrombotic events associated with aPL might occur in any vascular bed. On the other hand, the most common obstetric manifestation of the APS is RM, which is usually defined as three or more consecutive miscarriages before the tenth week of gestation. Thus, women with aPL are considered to be at increased risk for both RM and thrombotic events.

The aPL frequently persists for many years, possibly a lifetime without apparent harm. On the other hand, aPL antibodies can be detected in the sera of asymptomatic subjects even years before developing a full-blown disease. Thus, an unresolved critical question is what additional factors lead to the sudden development of thrombosis, which occurs only in a minority of patients with these antibodies.

A "2 hit hypothesis" has been proposed to explain the clinical observation that thrombotic events do occur only occasionally, despite the persistent presence of aPL. The first hit (aPL) would increase the thrombophilic risk and a second hit is required so that the clotting takes place. Interestingly, two short communications suggested, for the first time, a high incidence (59% of nonaspirin treated and 10% of aspirin treated patients in the study published by Erkan et al. (2001) and 3.8% of aspirin treated patients in the Tincani et al.'s (2001) study) of nonpregnancy-related vascular thrombosis in APS patients who present with pregnancy loss (i.e., the second hit) as their only manifestation of APS. One of these reports, however, was a retrospective data collection including a total of 65 patients of whom 50% were receiving aspirin therapy, while the second report was a cohort study including 52 women treated with aspirin. The results of these studies suggested that there is a high incidence of subsequent thrombosis in APS patients who present only with pregnancy loss and that aspirin may be indicated for thrombosis prophylaxis in this subgroup. However, thromboembolic events can occasionally be observed also in APS patients treated with low-dose aspirin. Other authors have also suggested that a history of RM in APS patients is a risk factor for subsequent thrombosis in the long term. In this report, however, both idiopathic and APS-RM patients were associated with a similar long-term risk of thrombosis. Nevertheless, in that study congenital or acquired thrombophilia other than aPL were not excluded and patients with one or more fetal deaths beyond 10 weeks gestation were included in the same group as women with three or more miscarriages before 10 weeks gestation.

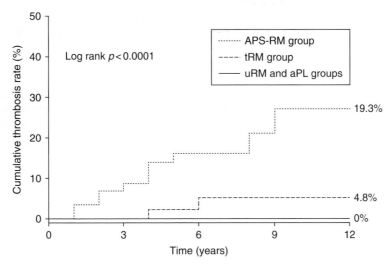

Figure 14.1 Kaplan–Meier curves of 12-year cumulative incidence of thrombotic events in four groups of patients studied by our research team: aPL group, women with positive tests for antiphospholipid antibodies (aPL) without pregnancy or thrombotic morbidity (laboratory testing for aPL was performed at the time of patients attending our hospital); APS–RM group, antiphospholipid syndrome patients with recurrent miscarriage; tRM group, patients with RM without aPL but with other known thrombophilias; uRM group, patients with RM without aPL or other known thrombophilias.

In a recent study performed by our group, Martínez-Zamora *et al.* (2012) have investigated whether patients with APS (all patients tested positive for aPL on three or more occasions at least 12 weeks apart, patients with lupus anticoagulant, medium to high levels of immunoglobulin (Ig)G and/or IgM anticardiolipin antibodies, or both, were included and those with only low IgG and/or IgM anticardiolipin antibodies were excluded) as the only etiological factor for RM are at increased risk of thrombosis later in life and have added new relevant information from a clinical point of view, showing that patients with RM associated with the presence of aPL have an increased long-term risk of thrombosis. This study used appropriate control patients (idiopathic RM patients, RM patients with thrombophilic genetic disorders, as previously described (please see the section "Are nonpregnant women with a history of RM in a prothrombotic state?"), and healthy aPL positive women without obstetric or thrombotic complications). There was statistically significant difference in the rate of thrombosis in the APS group compared with the three control groups (Figure 14.1). The rate of thrombosis was similar in idiopathic RM patients and aPL negative RM patients with genetic thrombophilias. Patients in the APS group had 25.6 thrombotic events per 1000 patient-years (95% CI 12.8–45.9) while the corresponding figure in the genetic thrombophilia group was 7.1 thrombotic events per 1000 patient-years (95% CI 0.8–25.5). The OR of thrombosis in relation to the presence or absence of aPL in patients with RM was 15.06 ($p < 0.0001$). This was still true when only patients with thrombophilic disorders other than aPL were considered (OR 4.8; 95% CI 1–22.8) ($p < 0.05$). Accordingly, the OR was even higher when the APS-RM group was compared with the idiopathic RM group alone (OR 42.8; 95% CI 2.5–742) ($p < 0.0001$).

Remarkably, 71.4% APS-RM patients who were diagnosed with arterial thrombosis had concomitant thrombosis risk factors (hypertension, hypercholesterolemia, and smoking).

> ** ⚒ SCIENCE REVISITED**
>
> The presence of circulating aPL rather than thrombophilic genetic defects in patients with RM is a determinant of thrombotic events later in life, especially among those aPL-positive RM patients also having cardiovascular risk factors.

Interestingly enough, only 19.3% of APS-RM patients and no woman among the healthy aPL positive women developed a thrombotic event in the long-term, despite aPL and aCL and their isotype distribution being similar in aPL-positive patients developing thrombosis or not and irrespective of being RM or healthy controls.

Moreover, the occurrence of thrombotic events among aPL-positive women with RM treated with low-dose aspirin was not different than in patients who did not receive this treatment (OR 2.9; 95% CI 0.5–15.1). However, the latter cannot be definitely concluded in this study, given the low number of subjects treated with low-dose aspirin and the fact that the treatment was arbitrarily administered according to the physician's criteria.

In conclusion, this recent study suggests that a history of RM associated with aPL is a risk factor for subsequent thrombosis in the long term. Moreover, thrombosis in APS-RM patients is frequently associated with concomitant cardiovascular risk factors.

Should Patients with Previous RMs Receive Thromboprophylaxis in the Long-term?

The limited available data in the literature do not justify yet the use of thromboprophylaxis in idiopathic RM patients. Nevertheless, according to previous studies which suggest long-term risk of arterial events in RM individuals, patients should be advised to avoid traditional cardiovascular risk factors and physicians should individualize the risk.

Furthermore, genetic thrombophilias such as Factor V Leiden and prothrombin mutations are widely accepted in daily clinical practice as a cause of RM and thus, thromboprophylaxis is used in the next pregnancy in these patients. This notwithstanding, some authors question this approach. The use of thromboprophylaxis later in life after pregnancies in RM patients with genetic thrombophilias and no previous thrombosis, is, generally, not recommended. However, similarly to idiopathic RM patients, RM patients with genetic thrombophilias may benefit from counseling about avoiding cardiovascular risk factors.

Nowadays there is no way to predict when or which healthy aPL patients will develop thrombosis. However, the presence of circulating aPL rather than thrombophilic genetic defects in patients with RM is a determinant of thrombotic events later in life, especially among these APS-RM patients with cardiovascular risk factors. The aforementioned notwithstanding, in this respect, several studies suggest that aPL-positive individuals should be risk-stratified according to traditional cardiovascular risk factors, which can be responsible for triggering acute thrombosis. It may seem that treatment and/or prevention of these thrombosis risk factors could be an important intervention to reduce arterial thrombosis. Thus, there is support to the "2 hit hypothesis" where aPL (which would be the "first hit") increases the thrombophilic risk and the clotting takes place in the presence of another thrombophilic condition (i.e., RM associated with traditional cardiovascular risk factors or not, acting as the "second hit"). This would explain previous epidemiologic studies suggesting that a woman's reproductive history may indicate future cardiovascular risk. On the other hand, it is to note that, as for other autoimmune diseases, the etiopathogenesis of APS is also apparently multifactorial, involving responses of both adaptive and innate immunity, being supported by a genetic background and triggered by environmental factors. In other words, genetically determined and environmental factors (second hits) may cooperate with aPL (first hit) in favoring thrombotic events. Therefore, whether an individual will develop a thrombotic event will depend on the concomitant presence of additional factors that may increase the whole thrombotic risk. This would explain why up to 80% of patients with RM associated with aPL did not develop a thrombotic event.

The earlier-discussed facts may have clinical implications regarding prophylactic antithrombotic therapy, mainly in those aPL-positive and RM patients with cardiovascular risk factors. The efficacy of long-term thromboprophylaxis and its associated risk of bleeding is a complex problem in aPL-positive patients who have not developed previous thrombosis, or in APS patients with isolated obstetric morbidity. While most authors advocate the use of antithrombotic therapy only in patients with aPL and thromboembolic events, there is no consensus as to whether patients who have not yet experienced any thrombotic event might also be given prophylaxis. A retrospective observational study has suggested that low-dose aspirin may be effective in the prevention of thrombosis for asymptomatic, persistently aPL-positive individuals who have additional thrombosis risk factors APS. Moreover, a recently published prospective study found that hypertension and lupus anticoagulant were independent risk factors for thrombosis in aPL carriers, and therefore recommend the use of thromboprophylaxis in these subjects and limited to high-risk situations. For patients with RM and aPL, this issue cannot be solved by the scanty, incomplete, and contradictory data resulting from the studies previously reported in the literature. Thus, further studies are warranted to assess the efficacy and risks of long-term thromboprophylaxis with low-dose aspirin and/or heparin in patients with RM associated with aPL.

Bibliography

Cervera, R. and Balasch, J. (2008) Bidirectional effects on autoimmunity and reproduction. *Human Reproduction Update*, **14**, 359–366.

Erkan, D., Merrill, J.T., Yazici, Y. *et al.* (2001) High thrombosis rate after fetal loss in antiphospholipid syndrome: effective prophylaxis with aspirin. *Arthritis & Rheumatism*, **44**, 1466–1467.

Martínez-Zamora, M.A., Peralta, S., Creus, M. *et al.* (2012) Risk of thromboembolic events after recurrent spontaneous abortion in antiphospholipid syndrome: a case-control study. *Annals Rheumatic Diseases*, **71**, 61–66.

Rai, R. (2003) Is miscarriage a coagulopathy? *Current Opinion in Obstetrics Gynecology*, **15**, 265–268.

Smith, G.C.S., Pell, J.P. and Walsh, D. (2001) Pregnancy complications and maternal risk of ischaemic heart disease: a retrospective cohort study of 129290 births. *Lancet*, **257**, 2002–2006.

Tincani, A., Taglietti, M., Biasini, C. *et al.* (2001) Thromboembolic events after fetal loss in patients with antiphospholipid syndrome. *Arthritis & Rheumatism*, **46**, 1126–1127.

How to Organize and Run an Early Pregnancy Unit/Recurrent Miscarriage Clinic

AnnMaria Ellard and Roy G. Farquharson

Miscarriage Clinic, Liverpool Women's Hospital, Liverpool, Merseyside, UK

Introduction

The recent appearance of early pregnancy units (EPUs) in the United Kingdom has moved quickly and seamlessly from innovation to routine clinical practice in the absence of evidence-based assessment or health economic analysis. Whether this process has followed an intuitive path fuelled in part by patient demand and management efficiency savings remains unanswered. Nevertheless, the fact that over 200 units are in active existence makes clinical sense that attracts ever-increasing demand allied to an enthusiastic adoption by trained healthcare professionals. The appearance of identical units in the Netherlands and other European Union countries is testament to their need and popularity.

Early pregnancy problems form a major part of all gynecological emergencies. Less common acute gynecological emergencies include acute collapse, suspected malignancy, and ovarian cyst accidents. All women with early pregnancy and acute gynecological problems should have prompt access to a dedicated EPU that provides efficient, evidence-based care with access to appropriate information and counseling. The National Service Framework recommends that all women should have access to an EPU that should be easily available (earlypregnancy.org.uk/FindUsMap.asp). Ideally, these services should also be directly accessible to general practitioners.

A report of the National Confidential Enquiry into Patient Outcome and Death in 2011 states that when a patient with an acute healthcare problem arrives in hospital, he or she requires prompt clinical assessment, appropriate investigations, and institution of a clear management plan. There should be early decision making to include involvement of relevant specialties and other required services followed by timely review by an appropriately trained senior clinician. This should be undertaken in an environment that best matches their clinical needs. Although there is conflicting evidence on the optimal location for the assessment of emergency admissions, it has been recommended that these patients should undergo initial assessment in dedicated Emergency Assessment Units (EAUs). The rationale for the use of EAUs is that they can reduce both the emergency department workload and in-hospital length of

Recurrent Pregnancy Loss, First Edition. Edited by Ole B. Christiansen.
© 2014 John Wiley & Sons, Ltd. Published 2014 by John Wiley & Sons, Ltd.

stay. Patients can be seen sooner by a senior doctor, which will result in earlier decision making and so expedite treatment. This may improve patient outcome and satisfaction. Standards set by the Society for Acute Medicine state that there should be a designated lead clinician and clinical manager in charge of an EAU.

EPUs should be encouraged to work collaboratively to share good practice and participate in clinical audit and research to improve standards of care for all women with problems in early pregnancy. Feedback from support organizations such as the Miscarriage Association, The Ectopic Pregnancy Trust and the Association of Early Pregnancy Units (AEPU) suggests that patients want prompt and sensitive treatment of early pregnancy problems as well as a full explanation of management choices, which should be supplemented with easy-to-read patient information leaflets.

In the past, patients were admitted to the emergency-receiving ward and waited for a considerable length of time before undergoing ultrasound scan and clinical assessment. With the appearance of EPUs, an increasing number of women are being assessed and managed as outpatient or office attenders. The advent of high-resolution transvaginal ultrasound coupled with the improved access to serum hCG measurements has allowed the development of models of care and improved delivery of care.

Within the United Kingdom, the number of EPUs has increased to the extent that over 200 active units are registered with the AEPU. The AEPU has set out, since it is inception in 2001, to improve the standards of early pregnancy care and to provide a clearer pathway of the patient journey (earlypregnancy.org.uk/index.asp). At all times, women should be supported in making informed choices about their care and management. Easy-to-read information leaflets should supplement these choices. Appropriate follow-up systems should be in place to facilitate repeat scans or blood tests.

In recent years, ultrasound diagnosis and improved understanding of problems related to early pregnancy have led to the introduction of medical and expectant management of miscarriage and selected cases of ectopic pregnancy. Randomized controlled trials have provided evidence-based practice (rcog.org.uk/womens-health/guidelines). Patient choice has emerged as a powerful selector for treatment. The mission statement from the AEPU has the patient at the center of all activity and the multidisciplinary care structure reflects the multitasking approach of care providers. The recent publication by National Institute for Health and Care Excellence (NICE) (2012) on Ectopic Pregnancy and Miscarriage is a welcome addition.

All women with early pregnancy problems should have prompt access to a dedicated Early Pregnancy Assessment Unit (EPU) that provides efficient evidence based care with access to appropriate information and counseling. At all times women will be supported in making informed choices about their care and management.

Setting the scene

Within the United Kingdom, there are approximately 700 000 births, 200 000 terminations of pregnancy, more than 250 000 miscarriages, and 15 000 ectopic pregnancies per annum (1, CEMACE report, 2011). Added to this huge activity profile, there are clear trends and shifts that include the effects of increasing maternal age, increasing demand and access to acute gynecological services, increasing knowledge about early pregnancy events (approximately 17 500 000 entries on Google), and improved choices for patients of care provider.

Standards of practice

The opportunity is now here for clear core standards to be applied to harmonize care provision across the United Kingdom. As a consequence, the AEPU constructed 10 key points to lay down a solid foundation for care providers (CMACE) (earlypregnancy. org.uk/index.asp). In conjunction with the RCOG and patient groups including the Miscarriage Association, Ectopic Pregnancy Trust as well as related professionals especially psychologists, a set of standards has been published on early pregnancy care, ectopic pregnancy, and recurrent miscarriage. The importance of early pregnancy events and their subsequent impact on obstetric outcome is well documented.

STANDARDS FOR EARLY PREGNANCY UNITS

Patient Focus

Women should be offered a range of management options with a full explanation of the processes involved
There should be appropriately furnished room for breaking bad news
All emotional and psychological counseling requirements should be provided within the EPU
There should be access to bereavement counseling
Clear patient information should be available on pathology tests, postmortem examination, and sensitive disposal options

Accessibility

All units should offer a minimum service that includes a 5-day clinic opening during office hours, with full staffing and scan support. Ideally, there should be a 7-day service
There should be direct referral for women with a history of recurrent pregnancy loss or previous ectopic pregnancy

Environment

All units should have a designated reception area constantly staffed during opening hours
There should be direct referral access for other healthcare professionals such as accident and emergency departments, NHS Direct / NHS24

Process

All units should offer a full range of options for managing both miscarriage and ectopic pregnancy (conservative, medical, and surgical). Care pathways should be in place for each management option
Guidelines and algorithms should be in place for the management of:

- Pregnancy of uncertain viability
- Pregnancy of unknown location
- Suspected ectopic pregnancy

All units should have laboratory access to serum human chorionic gonadotrophin (hCG) measurement and blood group result available the same day. Ideally, blood group results should be available within 2 h

All women undergoing surgical intervention for miscarriage should be offered screening test for *Chlamydia trachomatis*

Access to daily serum progesterone assay as part of a clinical algorithm will facilitate management of cases of pregnancy of unknown location

Audit

All units should have regular clinical governance meetings to review clinical protocols, critical incidents, and to assess the need for continuing training

Staffing and Competence

All units should hold a register of staff competent in transabdominal and transvaginal scanning

All staff should undergo formal training for emotional and psychological support

Auditable Standards

All units should audit patient choice and uptake rates for medical/surgical/ conservative management of miscarriage, together with complications and failure rates

All units should audit on an annual basis adherence to the RCOG Green-top Guideline No. 25: *The Management of Early Pregnancy Loss*

Early pregnancy loss

Diagnosis

The diagnosis of miscarriage is based on a well-recognized, peer-reviewed protocol as summarized in Figure 15.1. Ultrasound diagnosis is used universally in the presence of an intrauterine sac and is confirmed by serial observation wherever doubt exists as to the viability of the pregnancy (PUV, pregnancy of uncertain viability). A second ultrasound trained observer should confirm the diagnosis of fetal loss (loss of previously documented fetal heart activity). Recent evidence suggests a minimum crown rump length of over 6 mm and a mean gestational sac diameter of more than 25 mm are minimum requirements before a validated diagnosis of pregnancy loss can be confidently made. If any doubt exists, a second scan should be repeated later by at least 1 week or more. In addition, there is a small risk, approximately 1 in 1000, that a misdiagnosis of early pregnancy loss may occur, especially at the very early stages using the aforementioned definition. Many patients in this situation request a subsequent scan to confirm the original finding and their request should be supported.

Management of early pregnancy loss

In recent years, ultrasound diagnosis and improved understanding of problems related to early pregnancy has led to the introduction of medical and expectant management of miscarriage and selected cases of ectopic pregnancy in addition to

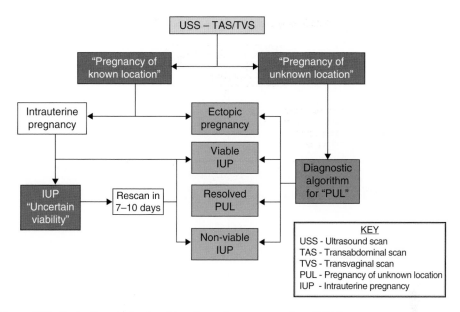

Figure 15.1 Basic diagnostic algorithm for early pregnancy loss (2006).

the traditional surgical option (Figure 15.2). Randomized controlled trials have provided evidence-based practice provided in the 2012 NICE guideline (NICE (2012)).

Patient choice has emerged as a powerful selector for the treatment of miscarriage. The mission statement from the AEPU has the patient at the center of all activity and the multidisciplinary care structure reflects the multitasking approach of care providers.

The drugs used for medical management of a miscarriage may include an antiprogesterone, oral mifepristone (200 mg), but always a prostaglandin such as misoprostol per vaginum or orally (200 µg×2 or 400 µg×2).

The original prostaglandin E_1 analogue used was gemeprost, and is effective in 95% of cases in combination with mifepristone at <63 days of amenorrhea. The alternative E_1 analogue, misoprostol may be given orally or vaginally and is most effective if administered vaginally (95% vs. 87%, respectively). The main advantages over gemeprost are that it does not require refrigeration; it is cheaper and can be administered orally or vaginally.

Contraindications to medical management

Absolute: Adrenal insufficiency
Long-term glucocorticoid therapy
Hemoglobinopathies or anticoagulant therapy
Anemia (hemoglobin <10 g/dl)
Porphyria
Mitral stenosis
Glaucoma
Nonsteroidal anti-inflammatory drug ingestion in previous 48 h
Relative: Hypertension
Severe asthma

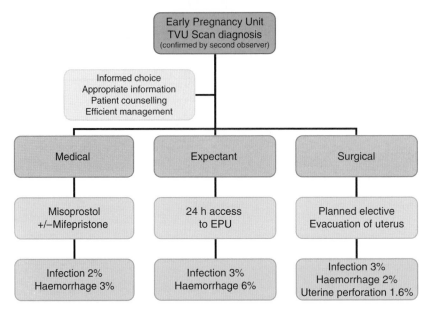

RCOG early pregnancy loss guideline 25, 2006

Figure 15.2 Management of miscarriage.

Varying rates of efficacy have been quoted with medical management in nonviable pregnancies. The efficacy is greatest for those pregnancies of less than 10 weeks or with a sac diameter of less than 24 mm (92–94%).

Protocol for medical management of miscarriage

- Ensure that the patient has read information leaflet
- Ask if she has any questions
- Follow local EPU protocol
- Obtain written consent for mifepristone and misoprostol administration
- Arrange blood tests
  - Measurement of hemoglobin concentration
  - Determination of ABO and Rhesus blood groups with screening for red cell antibodies
- Anti-D immunoglobulin should be given to all nonsensitized RhD-negative women undergoing medical evacuation.
- In the case of a pregnancy occurring with an intrauterine contraceptive device in-situ, the device should be removed before administration of mifepristone.
- Prescribe mifepristone 200 mg orally.
- Arrange attendance 24 (24–72) h after mifepristone administration.
- Inform the patient regarding the length of stay. Observe for 3 – 6 h after administration of prostaglandin and discharge if clinically well.
- Women with gestation:
  - <9 weeks on scan can have only one insertion of misoprostol 800 µg vaginally. Misoprostol tablets are administered vaginally, either by the woman herself or

the clinician. If miscarriage has not occurred 4 h after administration of misoprostol, a further dose of misoprostol 400 µg may be administered orally or vaginally.

- ○ >9 weeks on scan can have a maximum of four further doses of misoprostol 400 µg at 3-h intervals, vaginally or orally depending on the amount of bleeding and patient's preference.
- Prescribe prostaglandin (misoprostol 800 µg tablets/cervagem 1 mg) vaginally and metronidazole 1G rectally on the drug chart.
- Prescribe pain relief after the procedure.
- Inform that in case of heavy bleeding surgical management may be required and therefore she should be prepared to stay overnight if necessary
- Women may or may not pass "miscarriage tissue" while on the ward. They should be advised of what to expect when they go home and not referred to EPU for a scan before their follow-up appointment as most of them would miscarry at a later stage after discharge from the hospital.
- Any tissue that is obtained should be sent for histological examination to exclude a molar pregnancy or arrange a urine pregnancy test 3–4 weeks later.
- Give patient information on:
  - ○ Admission to gynecology ward
  - ○ Medical management of nonviable pregnancy
  - ○ What to expect and the likely amount of blood loss
  - ○ What analgesics to be taken
  - ○ What sort of sanitary protection to be used
- Arrange follow-up in EPU *3* weeks later and check urine pregnancy test (so as to avoid further appointments if miscarriage tissue is seen at an early scan or a surgical intervention)
- Cancel any outstanding antenatal or ultrasound appointments
- Inform the general practitioner and community midwife so that they can provide ongoing support at home
- Give contact telephone numbers for EPU/Gynecology Emergency Room/Ward

Surgical management of miscarriage

Surgical evacuation should be preferably managed on a day-case basis unless there is heavy bleeding when the patient should be admitted urgently to gynecology ward.

Have a local unit protocol for admission system with a patient pathway clearly described.

Give the patient information on admission procedure including appropriate patient information leaflet(s).

Explain the surgical procedure and obtain written consent by a doctor familiar with the procedure. Mention rare anesthetic and uncommon surgical risks involved such as uterine perforation (1%), cervical tears, intra-abdominal trauma (0.1%), intrauterine adhesions, hemorrhage, and infection.

Arrange for measurement of hemoglobin concentration and determination of ABO and Rhesus blood groups. Anti-D immunoglobulin should be given to all non-sensitized Rh D negative women undergoing surgical evacuation.

All at-risk women (usually women under the age of 25 years) undergoing surgical evacuation for miscarriage should be screened for *C. trachomatis*. If Chlamydia infection is identified, women and their partners should receive antibiotics.

Routine antibiotic prophylaxis is not recommended prior to surgical evacuation.

Current recommendations are that all tissue obtained at a surgical evacuation for miscarriage should be sent for histology examination. The reasons are:

1. To diagnose molar pregnancy
2. To exclude ectopic if chorionic tissue is not found on histology

A follow-up appointment is usually not required after a surgical evacuation.

Give patient information on "What you may need to know after a miscarriage." There should be information on counseling if required in the future.

Expectant management of miscarriage

A significant number of women prefer expectant management and it may be continued as long as the patient is willing, provided there are no signs of infection such as:

- Vaginal discharge
- Excessive bleeding
- Pyrexia
- Abdominal pain

Conservative management requires:

- Motivation and preparation
- A thorough explanation on:
  - What to expect: the likely amount of blood loss and pain
  - What analgesics to be taken
  - What sort of sanitary protection to be used
- Satisfactory answers to their questions and doubts
- Reassurance that the risk of infection is negligible (<3%)
- A contact number should be available 24 h if there are any problems, such as very heavy loss or severe pain. An adequately informed and reassured patient is less likely to contact for any further advice.
- A follow-up appointment for confirmation that the miscarriage is complete and to assess if she has any pain or bleeding
- An information leaflet to support verbal explanation.

Success rates are higher with prolonged follow-up. Follow-up scans may be arranged at 2-weekly intervals, until a diagnosis of complete miscarriage is made. However, if patient requests a surgical or medical method at any stage, her request should be accommodated. In general, 90% of women miscarry in 3 weeks time. Only a small percentage of women may go up to 6–8 weeks.

In the absence of clinically different relevant differences in safety, noninvasive treatment modalities can now be offered with confidence to women with first trimester miscarriage who wish to avoid surgical evacuation. This is important since freedom of treatment choice improves quality of life in these patients. Infection rates (2–3%) after expectant, medical, and surgical management are not significantly different and are reassuringly low.

Ectopic pregnancy

As ectopic pregnancy is a life-threatening condition women should have prompt access to a dedicated EPU providing efficient management and patient counseling. EPUs should have a protocol in place for conducting a pregnancy test and transvaginal ultrasound in women of reproductive age with amenorrhea associated with abdominal pain Figure 15.3. Access to serial serum hCG (human chorionic gonadotrophin) laboratory measurements is mandatory for efficient diagnosis, surveillance, and monitoring. All units should have clear guidelines in place for the management of pregnancies of unknown location (PULs) (earlypregnancy.org.uk/guidelines).

The application of an algorithm for management of PUL, given later, is a useful start to the eventual diagnosis of ectopic pregnancy. The background prevalence of ectopic pregnancy is of the order of 3–10%, depending on the type of population studied and cohort analysis.

Recurrent miscarriage

Recurrent Miscarriage Clinics

Recurrent miscarriage (RM) is defined as three or more consecutive pregnancy losses and affects about 1% of couples. More particular definitions include three consecutive early pregnancy losses (empty sac type) or two consecutive fetal losses (loss of fetal heart activity following ultrasound confirmation). Maternal age and the number of previous losses are two of the most important factors in determining future prognosis. Although the pathophysiology remains unknown in almost 50% of cases, congenital uterine abnormalities and maternal thrombophilia have been directly associated with RM.

All RM clinics should have a clearly defined protocol for the investigation of women with RM (Figure 15.4). It is vital that patients should have preconceptual investigation and counseling and more importantly, easy access to the clinic for support and surveillance as soon as they see a positive urine pregnancy test in the next pregnancy. To improve care and provide a positive patient experience, the following diagram provides the essential elements for a patient-focused service (Figure 15.5). Patient communication and support is key to a successful caseload.

Following preconceptual assessment and counseling, many couples remain unaware of the future chance for success, especially for the majority who have no identifiable cause. The use of a prediction success matrix provides a reasonable basis for help and patient empowerment (Figure 15.6).

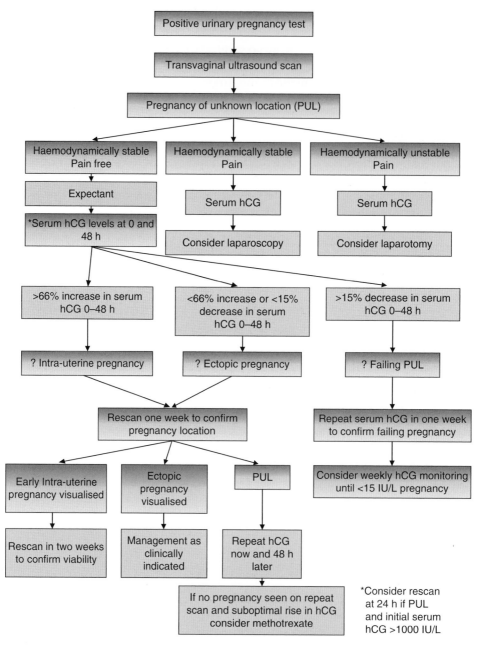

Figure 15.3 Suggested PUL algorithm for management of suspected ectopic pregnancy.

Staffing and training implications

It is accepted that only appropriately trained and competent staff should perform transabdominal and transvaginal early pregnancy scans. Sonographers, specialist nurses, and clinicians should aspire to produce ultrasound reports following standardized RCR/RCOG documentation. Postgraduate trainees need supervision from their educational

Miscarriage clinic: List of Investigations

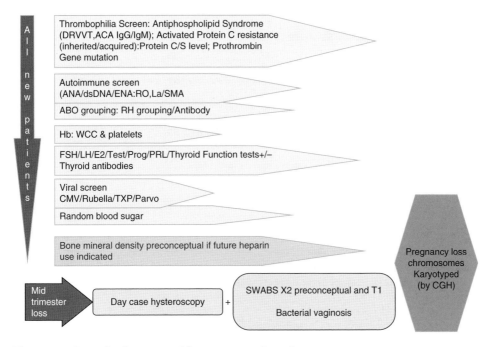

Figure 15.4 Investigation protocol for recurrent miscarriage.

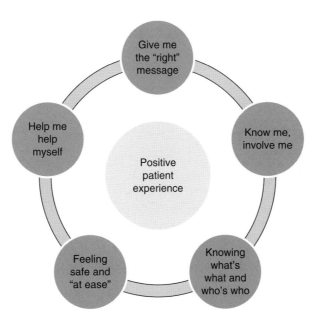

Figure 15.5 Positive patient experience.

Age	Number of Previous Miscarriages			
(yrs)	2	3	4	5
20	**92**	**90**	**88**	85
25	**89**	**86**	**82**	79
30	**84**	**80**	**76**	71
35	**77**	**73**	**68**	62
40	69	64	58	52
45	60	54	48	42

Following idiopathic RM, the predicted probability (%) of successful pregnancy is determined by age and previous miscarriage history (95% confidence interval <20% in bold).

Figure 15.6 Success prediction matrix for idiopathic recurrent miscarriage. Brigham SA, Conlon C, Farquharson RG. A longitudinal study of pregnancy outcome following idiopathic recurrent miscarriage. Human Reproduction 1999; 14: 2868–2871.

PEARLS TO TAKE HOME

Patient Focus

Information leaflets should be available for women and their families on local referral pathways, investigation, management, and future care.

All women with a history of RM should be offered a follow-up visit to discuss issues such as fertility and early management of subsequent pregnancies.

Accessibility

All women who present with known criteria for RM should be offered advice and referred to an EPU/specialist clinic either locally or at a tertiary unit.

Environment

All women with RM should have access to an EPU/miscarriage clinic with appropriately trained healthcare professionals.

Arrangements should be in place for women with a future confirmed pregnancy test to attend an EPU for an ultrasound scan and to receive shared antenatal care in a high-risk obstetric clinic.

Process

There should be a clearly defined protocol for investigating couples with RM.

Couples should be informed that women whose ovaries have a polycystic appearance at ultrasound scan and who ovulate are not at increased risk of RM and will not require antiestrogen treatment.

Three-dimensional ultrasound should be used for assessment of uterine malformations, as it may prevent the need for diagnostic hysteroscopy and laparoscopy.

Cervical weakness should be considered only in women presenting with recurrent mid-trimester loss.

Preimplantation genetic screening has no evidence base in the management of RM.

Each unit should have a care pathway in place for managing a diagnosis of recurrent mid-trimester loss as regards cervical cerclage and transvaginal assessment of cervical length.

Thromboprophylaxis should be commenced with aspirin, with or without heparin for women with antiphospholipid syndrome and thrombophilia from diagnosis of intrauterine pregnancy. Venous Thromboembolic Disease risk assessment should be performed in all cases. Heparin should be continued for 6–8 weeks postpartum, with bone mineral density surveillance.

Cytogenetic analysis of the products of conception should be considered for women who have undergone treatment in the index pregnancy or have participated in a research trial.

Audit and Outcome

All clinical staff should attend regular clinical governance meetings and a record should be maintained. Standard agenda items should include audit, adverse incidents, protocols, and service development.

Staffing and Competence

All RM clinics should have in place a named consultant with a special interest in RM.

All RM clinics should have multidisciplinary support from genetics, EPU, pathology, radiology, and hematology departments.

All staff dealing with RM should be trained in emotional aspects of pregnancy loss, to provide immediate support and to enable access to specialist counseling.

Auditable Standards

All services should audit, on an annual basis, adherence to the RCOG Green-top Guideline No. 17: *The Investigation and Treatment of Couples with Recurrent Miscarriage*

supervisor or lead clinician to ensure competency and observations of their skills in examination and scanning as part of their formative assessment of skills.

All RM clinics should have a designated lead consultant with a special interest in RM. In addition, all medical and nursing staff should undergo formal training in breaking bad news and training to provide emotional and psychological support.

Ideally, all gynecologists should be able to conduct laparoscopic surgery in the management of ectopic pregnancy. Trainees should in the future complete an advanced training skills module in early pregnancy and laparoscopic surgery.

Opportunities for specialist training

There are training courses now available to specialist trainees as they progress through their careers. It is recommended that trainees complete the modules of intermediate ultrasound in gynecology and intermediate ultrasound of early pregnancy complications, before embarking on the advanced training skills module in acute gynecology and early pregnancy.

Audit and research issues

As an essential component of clinical governance, all EPUs and RM clinics should have regular meetings to review clinical guidelines and protocols. This would provide an ideal opportunity to discuss audits and generate research ideas and to discuss recruitment to national or international multicenter trials.

Regular audits should be undertaken to include patient choice regarding management of miscarriage and ectopic pregnancy and associated complications

---

PEARLS TO TAKE HOME

All women with early pregnancy complications should be evaluated in a dedicated EPU

Management of patients should be conducted by trained and competent staff

Adequate facilities should exist to perform scans and for the measurement of serum β-hCG levels

Algorithms should be in place to guide management of sporadic and RM and ectopic pregnancy

Adherence to local and national standards should be audited regularly

---

PATIENT ADVICE

Patients should be offered informed choice of management options

Patients should be furnished with written information in nonmedical language

Bereavement counseling should be offered to all patients who suffer a pregnancy loss

---

☆ TIPS AND TRICKS

A quiet room conducive to breaking bad news should be located away from the work area and ideally with a separate exit door.

associated with the various methods. Units should specifically include the medical and surgical management of ectopic pregnancy and include percentage of laparoscopic management of ectopic, rates of ruptured ectopic pregnancies, and incidence of failed diagnosis of ectopic pregnancy.

It is highly recommended that patient surveys with regard to patient satisfaction with facilities and counseling are included in order to identify areas that need improvement.

Bibliography

Association of Early Pregnancy Units (AEPU), website: www.earlypregnancy.org.uk/index.asp (accessed 25 June 2013).

Brigham SA, Conlon C, Farquharson RG. A longitudinal study of pregnancy outcome following idiopathic recurrent miscarriage. *Human Reproduction, 1999*; **14**: 2868–71.

Centre for Maternal and Child Enquiries (CMACE). Saving Mothers' Lives: reviewing maternal deaths to make motherhood safer: 2006–08. The Eighth Report on Confidential Enquiries into Maternal Deaths in the United Kingdom. *BJOG* 2011, **118** (Suppl. 1):1–203.

NICE (2012) *NICE Guideline on Ectopic Pregnancy and Miscarriage: Clinical Guidelines, CG154,* www.nice.org.uk (accessed 25 June 2013).

16

How to Organize an Early Pregnancy Unit/Recurrent Miscarriage Clinic – American Perspective

Joanne Kwak-Kim,[1] Kuniaki Ota[2] and Ae-Ra Han[2]

[1] Reproductive Medicine, Department of Obstetrics and Gynecology, Department of Microbiology and Immunology, The Chicago Medical School at Rosalind Franklin University of Medicine and Science, Vernon Hills, IL, USA
[2] Reproductive Medicine, Department of Obstetrics and Gynecology, Department of Microbiology and Immunology, The Chicago Medical School at Rosalind Franklin University of Medicine and Science, Vernon Hills, IL, USA

Introduction

Recurrent pregnancy loss (RPL) is a common obstetrical complication. However, its management in general obstetrical clinics is often problematic due to their various demands for evaluation, management, and support. Since RPL is often regarded as infertility and indeed, a significant proportion of women with RPL have either subfertility or infertility, women with RPL are often referred to and managed at infertility clinics or high-risk obstetric units. In either case, the management tends to be suboptimal. The infertility clinics do not offer continuous care for second and third trimester, and high-risk obstetrical clinics do not provide early pregnancy care. Therefore, establishment of a special clinic for RPL is ideal, if the number of potential patients justify the special clinic.

In general medical practice, organizing a special clinic is mostly due to a specific clinical demand raised by a specific group of patients. The specialty clinics are designed to meet for diagnosis of problems, and instruction or remedial work in a particular activity. Prior to establishing a special clinic, thorough investigation of clinical demand, a physical plant, and human resources (healthcare providers, administrators and office clerks, etc.) should be made. RPL has multiple etiologies and approximately 50% of them remain unexplained with current recommended evaluations. Therefore, investigation for possible etiology(s) and management of RPL are often confusing. In addition, RPL is an emotionally traumatic experience similar to that associated with stillbirth or neonatal death. When patients visit a clinician's office, they are anxious and hopeless. However, neither psychological evaluation nor support is routinely provided for women with RPL. In this review, current practice pattern for RPL is reviewed and principles for establishing a RPL specialty clinic are

Recurrent Pregnancy Loss, First Edition. Edited by Ole B. Christiansen.
© 2014 John Wiley & Sons, Ltd. Published 2014 by John Wiley & Sons, Ltd.

discussed including patient flow management, multidisciplinary team approach for comprehensive care and a physical facility.

Patient population at RPL special clinic

RPL has been classically defined as the occurrence of three or more consecutive losses of clinically recognized pregnancies prior to the twentieth week of gestation (ectopic and molar pregnancies are not included). There is a general consensus that healthy women should not undergo extensive evaluation after a single first trimester or early second trimester miscarriage, given these are relatively common and sporadic events: miscarriage occurs in about 10–15% of clinically recognized pregnancies under 20 weeks of gestation. Often, the circumstances surrounding the first pregnancy loss are not well investigated due to an emergency situation and a reported low risk for a repeated pregnancy loss. The overall risk of miscarriage in the next pregnancy remains about 15% after one miscarriage, but rises to 17–31% after two consecutive miscarriages, and to 25–46% after three or more miscarriages. In addition, prevalence of possible etiologies is the same among the women with two, three, or four or more RPLs. Based on this and similar data, most experts initiate evaluation and treatment of RPL after either two or three consecutive miscarriages. Recently, the American Society for Reproductive Medicine defined RPL as two or more consecutive pregnancy losses.

Healthcare Providers

RPL is often associated with multiple etiologies. Additionally, a significant portion of patients have comorbid conditions such as psychological, emotional, or social problems. Therefore, a multidisciplinary approach can be an effective management strategy. Women with RPL are often managed by a general obstetrician, a reproductive immunologist or an infertility specialist in the United States. Often the investigation includes genetic study of the product of conception, anatomical, endocrine, infectious, immunological, and hematological evaluations.

Multidisciplinary Team Approach

A comprehensive assessment and treatment plan can be designed by the input of a multidisciplinary team, including reproductive specialists and other healthcare specialists (Figure 16.1). The initial evaluation will begin with a visit to a general obstetrician or a reproductive immunologist. If patients have infertility or subfertility, in conjunction with RPL, an infertility specialist (reproductive endocrinology and infertility) should be involved for patient care. Each patient is evaluated to establish a care plan specific for her individual needs, and based on her clinical and psychosocial demands, the scope of the multidisciplinary team is determined. When patients progress beyond the first trimester, the second and third trimester treatment is coordinated with a high-risk obstetrical team and a perinatologist.

Who Serves on the Team?

The clinic should be organized to perform efficient and prompt clinical communications among the highly specialized expertise across a number of medical specialties.

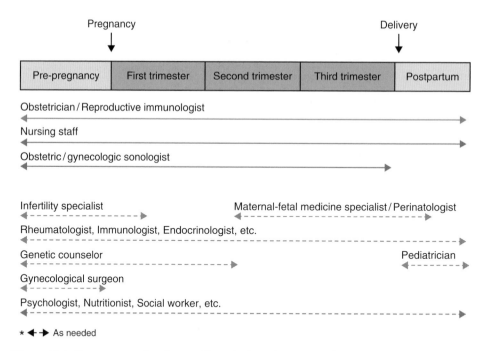

Figure 16.1 Engagement of patients with multidisciplinary team for prepregnancy, pregnancy, and postpartum management.

This "team medicine" approach helps ensure that diagnoses and treatment plans are personalized, and promotes better outcome for each and every patient. While there are no well-set guidelines, it is strongly believed that the RPL team should include an obstetrician, reproductive immunologist, reproductive endocrinologist, maternal fetal medicine specialist, nursing staff, genetic counselor, nutritionist, psychologist, and psychiatrist. Based on specific demands of RPL patients, some teams may include a rheumatologist, an immunologist, a hematologist, an endocrinologist, and/or an internist as well.

RPL teams are as diverse as the patients' demand. Teams also vary in their level of formality. Some make it a point to follow up on all cases that are discussed so that team members receive feedback on outcomes. Others perform only timely involvement without a complete follow through. The latter format is more cost effective and often adapted in clinical practice. Commonly, one or two reproductive immunologists or endocrinologists are employed by the RPL clinic. Other specialists are not directly employed to the RPL clinic but often associated with the healthcare system or medical insurance system. They serve as external consultants. Therefore, effective communication between the physicians in RPL clinic and external consultants is a key to success in a RPL team operation. Periodic communication via mail, fax or e-mail, and a regular meeting can facilitate communication. Electronic medical records (EMRs) allow sharing patient encounters, exchanging medical information between healthcare providers, and facilitate clinical practice. Nevertheless, communication, coordination, and decision adjustment among the specialists and patients are the major tasks to overcome.

Interprofessional approach

A special RPL program needs a complex interdisciplinary approach undertaking with a team of healthcare providers. RPL clinics in the United States often have a physician, a nurse, a laboratory assistant, and a receptionist, etc. For example, in my clinic, a nurse practitioner, a registered nurse, a certified medical assistant, two ultra sonographers, a secretary, and two receptionists are working together. Each profession provides different levels of care to women with RPL and supports each other's function. Since RPL special clinics are rare in the United States, often patients reside in remote locations from the clinic. For patients in remote locations, follow-up consultations are sometimes given through a phone consultation after the full evaluation. Other communications with patients are made through e-mail, web-based patient portals, phone, and fax. Nursing assistance for continuous communication is essential for remote patient care. Local patients are followed at the clinics regularly for physical check-up, ultrasound, and laboratory work as usual.

Roles of healthcare providers

- An obstetrician, who manages pregnancy and may perform surgical interventions such as vaginal delivery, cesarean section, amniocentesis, cervical cerclage, etc.
- An infertility specialist, who provides evaluation and treatments for endocrine disorders, infertility, and subfertility.
- A maternal-fetal medicine specialist, otherwise known as a high-risk obstetrician, who specializes in diagnosis and treatment of the high-risk pregnancies.
- An obstetric sonologist who has expertise in defining the fetal diagnosis and its severity, and guiding diagnostic and therapeutic procedures.
- A geneticist or genetic counselor, who focuses on prenatal diagnosis, prognosis, genetic counseling, and the procedures involved in prenatal diagnosis.
- A perinatologist, who counsels pregnant patients and family prenatally with respect to expectations and outcomes, and prepares to continue care for the baby after birth.
- A pediatric surgeon, who, in conjunction with the neonatologist, continues postnatal management of the fetal disease process and formulates the fetal treatment plan.
- Pediatric subspecialists, such as cardiologists, cardiothoracic surgeons, neurosurgeons, and urologists, etc.
- Other specialists: rheumatologist, immunologist, endocrinologist, gynecological surgeon, etc.
- Nursing staff handle daily communication with the patients and other nursing duties for clinical management.
- A nutritionist reviews the patients' nutritional intake, and establishes nutritional guidelines for the patients.
- A psychiatrist and psychologist provide psychological evaluation and treatment of the patients.
- A social worker provides social support for the patients.

> **★ TIPS AND TRICKS**
>
> **Clinic Operation**
>
> Provide ample time for visit.
>   Establish working flow to maintain efficient, professional, and personalized care.
>   Maintain clean and ample clinic space with adequate medical equipment.
>   Adapt health information technology that facilitates communication and provides information and decision support to clinicians.

> **PEARLS TO TAKE HOME**
>
> **Patient Management**
>
> Establish a special care team for each patient based on her needs.
>   Offer intensive multidisciplinary planning and counseling.
>   Maintain prompt and efficient communication between healthcare providers and patients.
>   Ensure strong individualization, with interventions customized to the particular patient.
>   Provide patient-centered education with treatment intervention.

How to manage patient flow at special RPL clinic?

Establishment of a patient flow chart significantly reduces delay in patient evaluation and treatment in special RPL clinic (Figure 16.2). Prior to the initial visit, patients can register via mail, e-mail, fax, or internet. Medical records are established when registration process is completed and the initial visit is scheduled. Registration is also an informational process and patients are acquainted with accounting and operational policies of the clinic. Prior to the initial visit, old medical records are collected and reviewed by the healthcare providers. Medical record review gives detailed information about patients' history, which is often missed when direct face to face discussion was made with a patient. Collected old medical records are either filed with the medical record, or scanned and attached to the patient's EMR. When patients make their first office visit, clinical evaluation is initiated. Clinical evaluation includes history taking, physical evaluation, laboratory evaluation, ultrasound evaluation and consultation, etc. Based on initial evaluation, the scope of RPL team is determined. Periodic meeting or communication should be established among the team members.

Utilization of EMR system facilitates communication among the healthcare providers and increases work efficiency. Typically, an EMR is accessed and updated by multiple healthcare providers to provide a longitudinal record of a patient's medical history. EMR systems manage the storage and retrieval of individual records with the aid of computers, often over a network, from multiple locations and/or sources. Additionally, EMR systems can reduce medical errors, increase physician efficiency and reduce costs, as well as promote standardization of care in the RPL special clinics.

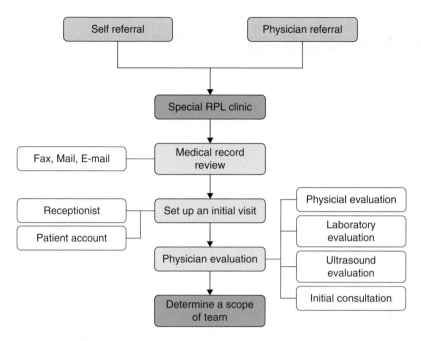

Figure 16.2 Patient flow algorithm at the special RPL clinic.

What to offer other than medical care?

In clinic organization, logistical, professional and quality assurance processes should be incorporated. Clinic should establish and offer the following to patients:

- maintain minimum/maximum number of patients they are willing/prefer to do each day
- fee per day or per management
- insurance coverage
- any preference on location if the clinic has multiple locations
- available dates over the next several months
- contract requirements
- how are travel and lodging expenses to be handled

Physical facility for the special RPL clinic

The necessary infrastructure for the support and maintenance of a RPL clinic facility should be carefully planned. When viewed functionally, a well-planned infrastructure facilitates the medical services, as well as basic social services at the clinic. The special RPL clinic area can be divided into three functional areas: areas for reception, clinical operation, and ancillary function (Table 16.1). A reception area provides patient registration, appointment, and accounting services. After registration process, patients are introduced to the area for clinical operation. The first entry point of the clinic area is a triage room. Vital signs and brief medical histories are taken by a nursing staff. After the initial assessment, patients are introduced to a physician at an exam room.

Table 16.1 Three Major Functional Areas in RPL Special Units

Functional area	Specific rooms or offices
Reception area	Reception with office functions (Fax, copiers, computers, and phones)
	Accounting services
	Patient waiting area
Clinic area for direct patient care	Triage room
	Physical exam room
	Procedure room
	Treatment room
	Consultation room
	Nursing station
	Nursing office
	Ultrasound unit
	Laboratory
Other ancillary functional area	Physician office
	IT room for computer and phone facility
	Medical record room
	Medical supply room
	Clean and dirty room facility
	Restroom
	Staff resting area
	Storage room
	Student/Fellow room (in educational setting)

Physical examination is performed and an in-depth history is taken by a physician. After the physician's evaluation, an initial consultation is given to the patient in regards to an evaluation plan. An examination room is equipped with an exam table and a sitting area for short discussion. A consultation room is often utilized for initial and follow-up consultations and patient education. A procedure room is needed for minor surgical procedures such as polypectomy or endometrial biopsy, etc. A medical treatment room is utilized for injection, infusion, or other treatment procedures. An ultrasound suite is one of the essential parts of the clinic where ultrasonographic evaluation of the patients is performed. A laboratory is employed for the collection of biological specimens for evaluation and follow-up testing of patients. After completion of the visit, patients are directed to the reception area for discharge, making a follow-up visit, or completing accounting issues.

Based on clinic setting, all specialists in the team can be either in the same office (often sharing the office on a part time basis) or in different offices. In either case, communication between "the team" should be assured. Patient encounters or formal letters from the healthcare providers can be circulated via mail, e-mail, or fax between the team members.

Ultrasound unit

Having an on-site ultrasound unit for women with RPL is an essential feature of the special RPL clinic. Since intense and frequent surveillances are made during the first trimester, on-site ultrasound evaluation allows immediate adjustment of current treatment plan and improves pregnancy outcome. Ultrasound evaluation includes two parts, one for structural developmental survey and the other for the vascular assessment. Ultrasound unit is usually equipped with two-dimensional ultrasound machines; however, 3D/4D ultrasound machines with Doppler capacity are also available.

Sonologists or ultrasound technologists should have in-depth knowledge of early human development, as well as an understanding of the complex nature of RPL, including psychological and emotional problems. Many women with RPL have a traumatic memory of ultrasound evaluation since the miscarriage news is often delivered while ultrasound evaluation is performed. Therefore, sonologists should be sensitive to patients' emotional response while ultrasound evaluation is performed.

Conclusion

Maintaining a high-quality RPL special unit requires keeping up with the latest innovations in reproductive medicine and technology while sharing open and caring communication with a patient and her partner. The team of healthcare providers must inform, educate, and obtain compliance to medical protocol to assure the best outcome for the patients. At the same time, the special RPL clinic is to guarantee the best possible patient care, while confronting the severe cost pressure, changing legal conditions, and the pressure of medical progress. RPL special clinics need to offer the highest possible level of care in an organized, cost-effective manner. It is hoped that the serious application of the principles outlined in this review will encourage the creation of many such successful clinics in the future.

Bibliography

Côté, M.J. 2000 Understanding Patient Flow. *Decision Line* (March 2000), pp. 8–10.

Kwak-Kim, J., Park, J.C. and Ahn, H.K. *et al.* (2010) Immunological modes of pregnancy loss. *American Journal of Reproductive Immunology*, **63**, 611–623.

Sills E.S., Perloe M. and Stamm L.J. *et al.* (2004) Medical and psychological management of recurrent abortion, history of postneonatal death, ectopic pregnancy and infertility: successful implementation of IVF for multifactorial reproductive dysfunction. A Case Report. *Clinical Experimental Obstetrics and Gynecology*, **31**(2):143–146.

17

Case Studies

Ole B. Christiansen[1,2]

[1]Unit for Recurrent Miscarriage, Fertility Clinic 4071, Rigshospitalet, Copenhagen, Denmark
[2]Department of Obstetrics and Gynaecology, Aalborg University Hospital, Aalborg, Denmark

Introduction

To work as a physician in a RM clinic can be distressing. Here I am not thinking about the distress and anger coming from seeing a patient suffering her seventh miscarriage after many years of struggle and failed attempts to get a child.

For a physician that really wants to base his/her managements on evidence-based medicine, it is distressing to acknowledge the fact that regarding RM, no test or treatment exists that are really evidence-based. As pointed out in Chapters 2, 6, 7, and 8, there is no real proof that surgical treatment of uterine anomalies, selection of embryos by preimplantation diagnosis (PGD) in case of parental aneuploidy, treatment of congenital thrombophilic disorders by anticoagulation, or treatment of immunological disturbances by allogeneic leukocyte or immunoglobulin (IvIg) infusions improve pregnancy outcome in patients with RM. The direct consequence that could be taken is that since there is no proven treatment for a detected risk factor, there is no need of screening for these factors.

Physicians and clinics with interest in RM can act in three different ways:

1. At one end of the spectrum are clinics such as the Amsterdam clinic (Chapter 2) that offers very few tests and treatments are only provided in the context of randomized-controlled trials (RCTs). This is of course the ideal situation seen from the aspect of the physician who wants all management to be evidence-based. The backside of this strategy is that its implementation requires very many resources in terms of money and manpower. Today, the performance of RCTs is, due to a huge amount of paperwork required for ethics committee approval, monitoring by good clinical practice units, applications for funding, etc., increasingly time-consuming. Pharmaceutical companies are in general reluctant to invest in research in RM, partly due to the heterogeneity of the condition and partly due to lack of centralization of RM management. To conduct good RCTs, there is a need for a big flow of patients to ensure that the trials are being finished within a reasonable time frame, but if the patients are offered only a minimum of investigations and only treatments in the context of RCTs, many will seek help

Recurrent Pregnancy Loss, First Edition. Edited by Ole B. Christiansen.
© 2014 John Wiley & Sons, Ltd. Published 2014 by John Wiley & Sons, Ltd.

elsewhere. Unfortunately, very few RM clinics possess sufficient manpower, lot of funding, and a big patient flow, and therefore high-quality studies in this area have been few.

2. At the other end of the spectrum are private clinics where treatments are paid by the patients themselves. Such clinics often offer screening programs that include almost every test that has been reported as being associated with RM in one of a few studies. In addition, in these clinics, a wide variety of treatments are being offered, often in combination, although no good documentation for the efficacy exists. These clinics will attract many patients, earn plenty of money, but will not provide any new knowledge about which investigations and treatments may be helpful in the management of RM.

3. In my clinic, we adhere to the pragmatic third point of view that we offer testing for a series of potential risk factors: uterine anomalies, parental chromosome aberrations, thrombophilia factors, autoantibodies, and maternal risk HLA-DR types. We recognize that no documented treatments exist in case of abnormal findings, but most of the factors have been proven to increase the risk of a further miscarriage and we primarily use the testing as a help for estimating the spontaneous prognosis and provide clarification for the patients. If no or few investigations are made, the patients will often invent their own, often undocumented, explanations for the miscarriages: some ingredients in the food, stress or noise at the working place, or some unspecified genetic mismatch with the husband, which may lead to malnutrition, loss of job, or divorce. If a screening program identifies one or two risk factors that exhibit a documented association to RM, this will often relieve the patients from self-blame and depression and encourage them to attempt pregnancy again, although the risk factors may not be directly treatable.

PEARLS TO TAKE HOME

Even though there is no direct treatment for a factor that has been demonstrated to be associated with RM or increase the risk of miscarriage (e.g., balanced chromosomal translocation, inherited thrombophilia factor, low plasma mannose binding lectin), its identification through a routine screening program for RM can often relieve the patient from self-blame and anxiety.

With regard to treatment, we have in my clinic only sufficient manpower and other resources to conduct one or two RCTs at a time – for the time being, a placebo-controlled trial of IvIg in patients with secondary RM and participation in a multi-center RCT, testing the efficacy of administering levothyroxine to euthyroid RM patients with antithyroid antibodies. All other patients are, after completing our screening program, being given an estimate of the spontaneous prognosis for live birth based on number of previous miscarriages, age, and results of the screening program. If the overall spontaneous chance for live birth is considered ≥50%, they are offered *tender loving care*: close monitoring with repeated plasma hCG and progesterone measurements until gestational week (GW) 6, and ultrasonic scans with intervals increasing from 1 to 2 weeks until GW16. If the spontaneous chance for birth is considered <50%, therapies with some documentation are offered; however, we clearly tell the patients that the documentation of the efficacy of the therapies is based on results from some trials whereas other trials have disagreed and that testing in RCTs is needed in the future. The treatment we offer to patients who cannot enter the RCTs is in most cases a combination of low-dose prednisone (10 mg daily) and IvIg (25 g at each infusion) from before conception, with continuation of IvIg infusions immediately after positive hCG, first weekly and later every second week until GW14 and continuation of prednisone to GW7 (see Chapters 6 and 7). This immunomodulatory treatment is offered relatively independently of finding or not finding immune disturbances in the blood since we recognize that immune disturbances displaying causal effects in RM may only be localized in the endometrium or uterine lymphoid glands. If plasma progesterone in early pregnancy is low or rapidly declining, we often advice vaginal progesterone supplementation, still telling the patients that the proof for the efficacy is based on small and old trials.

In the following, I will review the management of four patients from our clinic. The reproductive histories illustrate the dilemmas that physicians face when managing patients with RM and also exemplify how we in daily practice offer most patients with an estimated poor spontaneous prognosis of some kind of treatment, which is either in the context of a RCT or partly evidence-based. The case stories are not unique – each of them is representative for a group of patients with almost similar histories and outcome. The case stories can in my view illustrate some possible pathogenic pathways to RM and may stimulate new original thinking about causes of RM.

✋ CAUTION

Case stories cannot document the efficacy of any treatment

Case 1 is a woman who at the age of 30 had had two ultrasound confirmed miscarriages in GW7 followed by a miscarriage under a clinical picture of intrauterine fetal death in GW14. Karyotyping of the fetus by Achilles tendon biopsy revealed a normal fetal karyotype 46XX. Afterwards she had a pregnancy of unknown location (PUL). Her BMI was 35 and she had a menstrual cycle 35–40 days but endocrine screening did not support the suspicion of polycystic ovary syndrome (PCOS). Karyotyping of the couple showed that the woman carried a 46XX 16/17 karyotype, which is a balanced translocation between chromosome 16 and 17. Family investigation showed that the translocation was inherited from her father. She had a sister who also carried the translocation, who had given birth once and had no miscarriages. The husband's karyotype was normal 46XY but he was found to have decreased sperm quality. Investigation of the uterine cavity was normal.

At her local hospital, she was treated with metformin and underwent two trials of intrauterine insemination (IUI) with her husband's sperm but did not achieve pregnancy. Afterwards she was referred to an IVF clinic that attempted two trials of IVF with PGD. A total of five embryos were successfully cultured to the eight cells stage, allowing blastomere biopsies to be done, but all biopsies showed an unbalanced karyotype and no embryo transfer was undertaken. In 2004, she was referred to my clinic where thrombophilia screening was completely normal, immunological screening found her negative for a series of autoantibodies but the plasma level of mannose binding lectin (MBL) was only 3 µg/l. Previous studies from my group found that plasma MBL levels <100 µg/l are associated with an increased risk of RM and a 20% increased risk of miscarriage in the next pregnancy compared to patients with normal MBL levels. We therefore continued IUI with the husband's sperm in stimulated cycles but gave infusions of IvIg prior to each IUI resulting attempt. This resulted in two PULs in 2004.

Subsequently, we did not see the patient for more than a year but in 2006 she contacted us with a positive pregnancy test after spontaneous conception with the same husband. In the meantime she had lost some weight, now having a BMI of 30. We administered 11 infusions of IvIg from GW5 to GW20, and she gave birth to a girl by caesarean section due to breech presentation. The girl was healthy but carried the same balanced translocation as her mother.

The interesting message in this case history is that many RM couples display multiple risk factors for miscarriage, which may each contribute to the problem. In this case, the obvious risk factors were the patient's balanced chromosomal translocation, her overweight, her subfertility problem caused by the husband's low sperm quality, and lastly her low MBL plasma level. In other clinics, the focus was on the possible PCOS diagnosis and the chromosomal translocation. However, metformin treatment that can correct hyperinsulinemia and hyperandrogenemia in PCOS was not successful (see Chapter 8). The unsuccessful attempts of IVF with PGD emphasize the view provided in Chapters 2 and 6 that in couples with RM and a balanced chromosomal translocation, successful pregnancy will often be achieved more rapidly by spontaneous conception compared with IVF/PGD.

The fetus with normal karyotype miscarried in GW14 emphasizes the belief that the patient carries other risk factors for RM in addition to the chromosomal translocation. One of these factors may be the low plasma MBL level that may predispose to aberrant immune reactions toward the fetomaternal unit and cause especially late miscarriages. The combination of conceiving with an egg with a balanced translocation (by sheer luck), some weight loss, and IvIg treatment may have constituted the therapeutic cocktail responsible for the successful pregnancy outcome. However, the main issue is not to document whether any of the mentioned interventions may have been efficient or not, this cannot be done in a case report. The take-home message is that it is important to offer the full screening for risk factors to all RM patients and not halt investigations after identifying the first factor, for example, the balanced chromosomal translocation since competing risk factors will often be detected (see Chapter 5).

Case 1

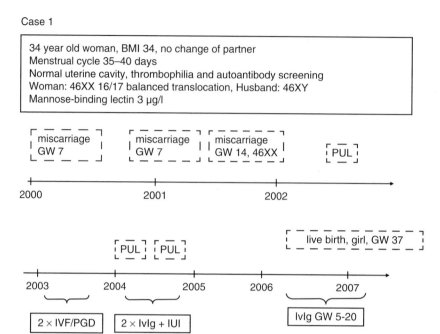

34 year old woman, BMI 34, no change of partner
Menstrual cycle 35–40 days
Normal uterine cavity, thrombophilia and autoantibody screening
Woman: 46XX 16/17 balanced translocation, Husband: 46XY
Mannose-binding lectin 3 µg/l

Case 2 is a woman who as a teenager experienced a chlamydial pelvic inflammation. In her first pregnancy at the age of 26 years, she had a ruptured tubal pregnancy resulting in left salpingectomy. After two spontaneously conceived PULs only confirmed by a positive plasma hCG measurement, she underwent ovulation induction with clomiphene citrate combined with metformin due to oligomenorrhea, hirsutism, and suspicion of PCOS. She conceived twice but again the pregnancies resulted in PULs. She now initiated IVF due to suspicion of tubal dysfunction (see Chapter 8). Prior to each IVF attempt, she was treated with contraceptive pills to ensure complete ablation of the endometrium before ovulation induction and also in order to suppress increased plasma and ovarian testosterone levels. She conceived twice in four IVF attempts but both pregnancies resulted in biochemical pregnancies. The patient was then referred to my clinic where she underwent screening for immunological and thrombophilic risk factors for RM. No autoantibodies were detected, but she had a low plasma MBL level of 30 µg/l and she carried the HLA type HLA-DR3 – both factors have in our previous studies been documented to be risk factors for RM and are associated with a decreased pregnancy prognosis in RM patients. We therefore offered her immunomodulatory treatment with a combination of prednisone and infusions of IvIg in the IVF cycle from before embryo transfer and continuing in the first trimester if pregnancy occurred. The first IVF cycle with immunomodulation was converted to IUI due to ovarian hyperstimulation, resulting in a PUL. In the next IVF cycle with immunomodulation, two embryos were transferred, a singleton intrauterine pregnancy was obtained and seven infusions of IvIg were provided until GW14. The pregnancy continued successfully and she gave birth to a healthy girl by caesarean section in GW35.

The messages that can be delivered by this case history are again that many RM patients have multiple risk factors for RM. In this case, suggested risk factors are PCOS/oligomenorrhea and generalized immunological hyperresponsivity suggested by the presence of MBL deficiency and carriage of the HLA-DR3 allele, both factors predisposing to a wide range of autoimmune diseases. An additional risk factor for early pregnancy loss was suspected tubal damage. It is possible, although it cannot be completely documented, that the PULs in the patient's non-IVF pregnancies had been spontaneously resorbed ectopic pregnancies localized in the right tube, which may have been damaged due to the previous chlamydial infection. The two biochemical pregnancies after IVF may have been a chance phenomenon since many IVF pregnancies end as biochemicals; however, it is also possible that they have been caused by harmful immunity acting very early after implantation and that the immunomodulatory treatment modified this dysfunction, resulting in the successful pregnancy. The main take-home message here is that more and more RM patients present with several PULs in the history. If an RM patient presents with a series of PULs, especially in the later part of the reproductive history, the differential diagnosis: repeated, spontaneously resorbed tubal pregnancies, should be considered and the patient may be referred for IVF (see Chapter 8).

Case 2

31 year old woman, BMI 25, no change of partner
Mestrual cycle 6–18 weeks
Normal uterine cavity, parental chromosomes, thrombophilia and autoantibody screening
Mannose-binding lectin 30 µg/l

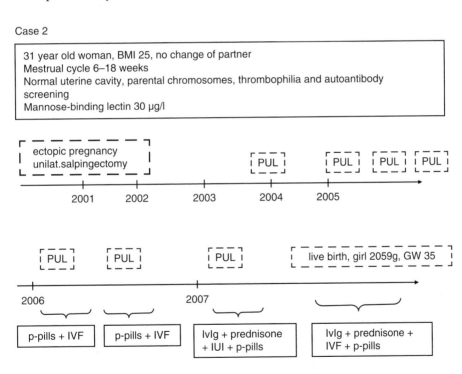

Case 3 is a woman who started her reproductive career at the age of 24. The first pregnancy ended with the intrauterine death of a normal but severely growth-retarded boy in GW22. Subsequently, she had two miscarriages prior to GW14 followed by another intrauterine death of a severely growth-retarded boy in GW20. At the first consultation in my clinic, she was healthy and had never experienced thromboembolic episodes. Our screening found that she was positive for the lupus anticoagulant and had titers of IgG anticardiolipin antibodies above the maximum detection limit. In her next pregnancy, she was treated with daily subcutaneous injections of low molecular heparin, low-dose aspirin and repeated infusions of IvIg until GW28. In GW28 she was, due to severe preeclampsia, delivered by caesarean section of a healthy but growth-retarded girl. One year after, she was again referred to my clinic with the wish of a second child and we gave her the same treatment as previously beginning from GW5. However, from GW23, heparin doses were increased to a daily dose of 10 000 IU due to suspicion of imminent intrauterine growth retardation, and due to severe preeclampsia, she was again delivered of a severely growth-retarded girl weighing 458 g by caesarean section in GW25. The girls survived in spite of extreme prematurity without significant sequela. In 2010, the patient was readmitted with a new husband and the wish of getting a third child. She received the same treatment as previously, although this time 10 000 IU of heparin was administered from GW8. However, in GW22, she developed severe preeclampsia and thrombocytopenia in spite of antihypertensive treatment and in GW22+5 intrauterine death of a severely growth-retarded girl was detected.

The message here is that all women with RM, but especially those with a history of second trimester miscarriage with or without high titres of antiphospholipid anti-bodies, are subject to a substantially increased risk of complications in the second half of pregnancy, often accompanied by severe preeclampsia and placental insufficiency in spite of up-to-date treatments with anticoagulation, etc. (see Chapter 11). A typical pattern seen in some of these patients is illustrated here; the disorder often worsens with age or parity and the pregnancies become severely affected at an earlier and earlier gestational age. This may emphasize the need for intervention in women with second trimester losses already after the second (or maybe the first late loss), since the disorder may worsen and become untreatable with increasing gravidity.

Case 3

26 year old woman, BMI 30, new partner last pregnancy
Mestrual cycle regular 30 days, healthy, no thromboembolic episodes
Normal uterine cavity, parental karyotypes and screening for non-antiphospholipid autoantibodies
Positive for lupus anticoagulant and IgG anticardiolipin >120 GPL-U/l

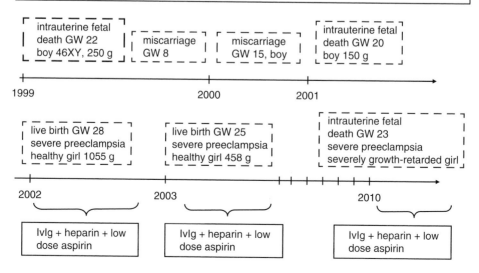

Case 4 is a woman who gave birth to a boy at an age of 28 years and afterwards she had had nine clinically documented first trimester miscarriages in spite of more and more extensive treatment attempts with heparin, IvIg, progesterone, and prednisone. All routine investigations were normal but the woman carried the HLA-DQ*0501 that have been proven to confer a reduced prognosis in women with secondary RM after the birth of a boy. The interesting message here is that only 1 year after the woman had gone though a completely uncomplicated pregnancy ending with the birth of a boy, she experiences the first of many subsequent miscarriages. The major circumstance changing from 2000 to 2001 is that she had carried a fetus and a placenta inside the uterus for 9 months. The risk of embryonal aneuploidy, endocrine disturbances, environmental risk factors etc. must be considered unchanged during the short period from 2000 to 2001. In my view, the most likely explanation for the rapid increase of miscarriage risk in this patient must be a change in her body occurring during her first pregnancy – most likely maternal immunization against proteins on the allogeneic fetus or trophoblast. Carriage of a pregnancy to the third trimester is associated with a well-known risk of development of maternal humoral or cellular immununologic reactions against fetal and placental proteins as seen in alloimmune immunization against fetal red cells or platelets. Our previous studies have provided evidence that maternal immunization against male-specific minor histocompatibility (HY) antigens may be a causal factor for secondary RM after the birth of a boy and is associated with a poor prognosis, especially in women with specific class II HLA alleles known to predispose to immunization against HY antigens such as HLA-DQ*0501. The case also illustrates that even when all traditional risk factors for RM: high age, subfertility, endocrine disturbances, autoantibodies, and thrombophilia, are absent, some women exhibit a very poor prognosis in spite of all available treatments. There is still room for identification of new causal factors for RM such as alloimmune reactions against major or minor histocompatibility antigens on the fetus or trophoblast.

Case 4

35 year old woman, BMI 31, no change of partner
Regular mestruations, no problems to conceive
Normal uterine cavity, parental chromosomes, endocrine, thrombophilia and
autoantibody screening. Normal mannose-binding lectin
HLA-DQB1*0501 positive

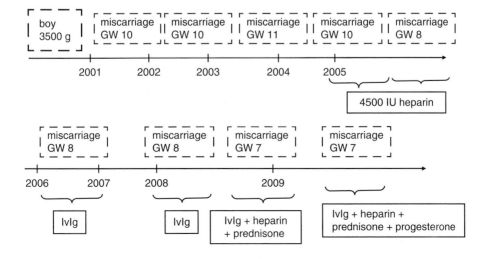

Overall, I must emphasize that these case stories do not provide any proof for the efficacy of any treatment for RM. The cases highlight (i) the fact that many couples with RM have multiple risk factors that should be identified if the problem is to be managed optimally, (ii) the fact that many pregnancy losses (PULs) may be ectopic pregnancies rather than miscarriages and should be treated accordingly, (iii) the fact that even if the pregnancy in an RM patient progresses to the third trimester, the risk of perinatal complications and death is substantial both in patients with and without the lupus anticoagulant, and (iv) the fact that some patients in spite of being negative for all recognized risk factors for RM exhibit a very poor pregnancy prognosis and may carry risk factors for RM that needs further clarification.

In conclusion, managing patients with RM is very challenging since the background of the different cases, as illustrated by the case stories, is very heterogeneous and treatments may only be efficient in subgroups with specific backgrounds. In addition, no or very few treatments have documented value. Testing treatments in RCTs can only be done in clinics with large patient flows, sufficient manpower, and in reality only in countries/areas where there are no competing clinics that offer treatments outside of RCTs since these will attract the patients.

Finally, research in RM including testing of treatments is complicated by the fact that pharmaceutical companies are reluctant to spend money on research in this area due to the heterogeneity of the condition, the lack of centralized management, and less focus on the condition in medical journals and at scientific congresses than "hot" topics such as stem cells, PGD, or ovarian freezing. International scientific societies with some focus on RM such as the ESHRE Early Pregnancy Special Interest Group or patient societies such as the British Miscarriage Association can hopefully increase the interest for this complex and distressing disorder, which is a prerequisite for getting sufficient resources allocated to the much needed testing of treatments in RCTs

Bibliography

Christiansen, O.B., Pedersen, B., Rosgaard, A. and Husth, M. (2002) A randomised, double-blind, placebo-controlled trial of intravenous immunoglobulin in the prevention of recurrent miscarriage: evidence for a therapeutic effect in women with secondary recurrent miscarriage. *Human Reproduction*, **17**, 809–816.

Empson, M.B., Lassere, M., Craig, J.C. and Scott, J.R. (2005) Prevention of recurrent miscarriage for women with antiphospholipid antibody or lupus anticoagulant. *Cochrane Database Systematic Reviews*, 2, CD002859.

Nielsen, H.S. (2011) Secondary recurrent miscarriage and H-Y immunity. *Human Reproduction Update*, **17**, 558–574.

Index

Recurrent Pregnancy Loss, First Edition. Edited by Ole B. Christiansen.
© 2014 John Wiley & Sons, Ltd. Published 2014 by John Wiley & Sons, Ltd.